Yoga
for
50+

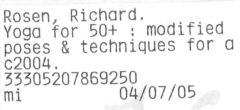
yoga

for 50+

Modified Poses
& Techniques
for a Safe Practice

Richard Rosen

photography by Robert Holmes

Published by: Ulysses Press
P.O. Box 3440
Berkeley, CA 94703
www.ulyssespress.com

Library of Congress Control Number: 2004101023
ISBN 1-56975-413-6

Printed in Canada by Transcontinental Printing

10 9 8 7 6 5 4 3 2 1

Copy Editors: Kathy Kaiser, Lily Chou
Editorial and production staff: Lynette Ubois, Steven Schwartz,
    Kaori Takee, James Meetze
Design: Sarah Levin
Photography: Robert Holmes
Models: Cathryn Yost, Clare Finn, George Lamb, Richard Rosen

Distributed in the United States by Publishers Group West
and in Canada by Raincoast Books

The authors have made every effort to trace copyright owners. Where they have failed, they offer their apologies and undertake to make proper acknowledgment where possible in reprints.

This book has been written and published strictly for informational purposes, and in no way should it be used as a substitute for consultation with health care professional. You should not consider educational material herein to be the practice of medicine or to replace consultation with a physician or other medical practitioner. The author and publisher are providing you with information in this work so that you can have the knowledge and can choose, at your own risk, to act on that knowledge. The author and publisher also urge all readers to be aware of their health status and to consult health professionals before beginning any health program, including changes in dietary habits.

Table of Contents

part one:

yoga basics

introduction

I turned fifty a few years ago. I didn't think much about it—that is, until the envelope arrived from the American Association of Retired Persons (AARP). Once you hit the half-century mark, Uncle AARP wants you. Uncle AARP's sudden interest in my age snapped me out of my complacency—or was it denial? Anyway, my first response was, *Me, retire? Not in this lifetime.*

Then I got to thinking about my yoga practice, and how my age had affected it. After some rumination, I realized that a couple of things about my practice or, more exactly, my body, had changed. I was a little stiffer, especially in the backs of my legs. I was also a little weaker: my handstands were quivering after only a minute when before I could hold on for two minutes or more. But my balance seemed okay, as did my endurance: I still started every practice session with fifteen to twenty rounds of Sun Salute.

The good news was that, after nearly a quarter-century of mostly regular practice, I was in touch with my body, including its intangible aspects. I might have been a tad looser and stronger when I was forty, but at fifty, I was a heck of a lot more intelligent about my body. My age had adversely affected my body to some degree, but my practice had very definitely softened the blow of advancing age. And I thought to myself, *Thanks, Yoga.*

You may believe that as you age, it's inevitable that your body won't work as well as it did ten or twenty years before, and there's some truth in this. But wait, all is not lost. Most experts agree that you *can* do something to counter the usual effects of aging, and that something is *exercise.* Just about any exercise, or combination of exercises, will work wonders. The only requirement is that you exercise regularly, at least four times a week, for about twenty minutes each time.

Unfortunately, just when you most need to get up and be active, you might shut down. *I'm too old*, you might think. Or (pick one), *I'm too heavy. It's too hard. I'm too fragile. I'm too weak. I'm too stiff. It's too boring. It's expensive. I'm too busy. I'm too tired.*

Typically, as we age, we become increasingly aware of, and try our best to avoid risky behavior. But studies suggest that one of the riskiest behaviors is *not* exercising. And it seems to me that yoga practice is particularly well suited to the task of keeping a person in peak condition.

Now, you might wonder whether a person in midlife needs a special book to teach him or her yoga. There isn't any reason that a fifty-year-old's practice has to be all that much different from a twenty-year-old's practice . . . eventually. At the start, though, you have to pace yourself more slowly than the average twenty-year-old, especially if you've been living a sedentary lifestyle, so that you don't overtax bones and joints, especially the knees, lower back, and neck.

The material in this book is basic, written with the beginner in mind. The book is divided into four parts, with an appendix tagging along at the end. Part I, this part, is like the foundation of a building: it contains information that you'll need to know before you get started, so please don't skip right to Part

II. Part II is like the foyer: its dozen simple exercises are an entranceway to the poses in Part III. Part III is the main room, consisting of about fifty poses, or asanas, many of them modified for beginners. Part IV puts the roof on the project, finishing with a couple of basic but essential breathing exercises. The appendix is like the house's decoration: it talks about how to sequence your practice, gives you some sequencing ideas, discusses how to keep yourself and your practice inspired over the long haul, and tells you how to find yourself the perfect yoga teacher.

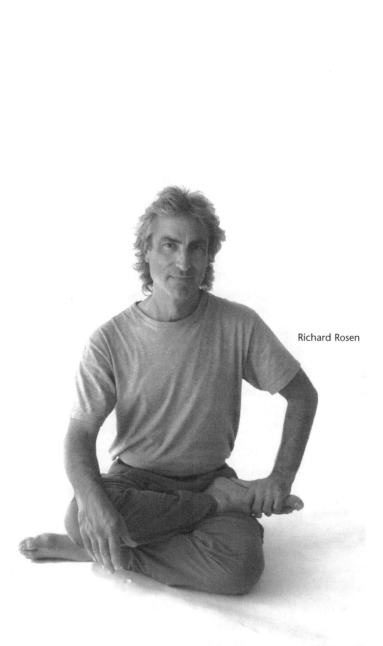

Richard Rosen

what is yoga?

The language of traditional yoga is Sanskrit. It's not spoken much nowadays, but once upon a time it was the tongue of India's educated elite. Sanskrit is an enormously evocative language, although not particularly easy to learn. But you should become acquainted with the Sanskrit names of the poses in this book; their meanings often provide hints about the subtler aspects of the poses.

Yoga is very old, two thousand years, at least. Tradition holds that the "father" of yoga is Hiranyagarbha (pronounced here-ahn-yah-gar-bah), Sanskrit for "golden seed." Western scholars tell us that Hiranyagarbha is likely a legendary character, and that yoga is probably the product of a group effort spanning several generations of practitioners.

The word *yoga* comes from the word *yuj*, "to yoke." This verb is the distant ancestor of a number of familiar English words, including *join*, *junction*, and *conjugal*. Although most Westerners equate yoga solely with the poses, or asanas, this is a misconception. There's actually no one practice you can point

to and say, *That's yoga*. Historically, there have been more than thirty distinct schools of yoga—most of them only marginally interested in asana, if at all. Some of them are still alive; others are extinct.

But whatever the school (even Hatha Yoga, the West's most popular form of yoga), yoga is essentially the practice of concentration training, or meditation: the persistent, methodical contemplation on the nature of the authentic self. This self isn't restricted to the mind, with its unceasing parade of thoughts, feelings, memories, fantasies, and so on. Yoga has a holistic view of the self that includes the body; the everyday "lower" mind; a "higher" mind, or insight-wisdom faculty (called *buddhi*, from *budh*, "to be awake"); and the *atman*, "soul."

The central question that all yoga meditation tries to answer is, *Who am I?*; or, if you flip the coin over, *How can I be truly happy?* The ultimate goal in most yoga schools is to realize the self's identity with, and then "yoke" it to, its Source, which the yogis call *Brahman*, the

"vast expanse." This may sound, at first, out of reach for the average person. But anyone who makes an honest effort will sample something of this lofty end.

Although the founders of traditional schools are often unknown or legendary characters (such as Hiranyagarbha), the founders of popular modern schools are widely known. Four of our most famous teachers are the students of one extraordinary man, a Brahmin Indian by the name of Tirumalai Krishnamacharya (1888–1989), whose work and teaching changed the face of yoga in the twentieth century. These teachers are Indra Devi (née Eugenie Peterson, 1899–2002), Sri Krishnamacharya's first female student, who opened the first yoga studio in the United States in Hollywood in 1947; B. K. S. Iyengar (b. 1918), Sri Krishnamacharya's brother-in-law and author of the modern classic *Light on Yoga*; K. Pattabhi Jois (b. 1918), the leading light of Ashtanga Vinyasa Yoga; and T. K. V. Desikachar (b. 1938), Sri Krishnamacharya's son, and the originator of Viniyoga.

general benefits of yoga

Yoga is, first and foremost, a *spiritual* practice. But the practice has a number of physical benefits. One text from the fourteenth century asserts that through yoga the body becomes lean and "glows" (*Hatha-Yoga-Pradipika* 2.19), the countenance becomes serene and the eyes clear, and the "fire" in the belly is stoked (*Hatha-Yoga-Pradipika* 2.78), improving digestion. A text from the seventeenth century says that yoga cures all kinds of diseases, and parries the sting of old age (*Gheranda-Samhita* 3.99).

We need to take the claims of traditional texts with a grain or two of salt, but modern research into yoga practice shows that the work has remarkable preventive and therapeutic possibilities. In fact, the field of yoga therapy is gaining mainstream acceptance as a treatment modality for various physical aches and pains. And one of the nice things about yoga is that, once you've gained some experience with the practice, you'll be able to actively participate in your own healing process. (For more information on yoga therapy, see the website of the International Association of Yoga Therapists at www.iayt.com.)

It's safe to say that *regular* practice will help to decelerate the aging process, both physically and psychologically. It's also been demonstrated that yoga can help ward off midlife health problems, including arthritis, osteoporosis, and low back pain. The yoga asanas help keep the jelly donut—like disks of the spine supple and improve posture. You might get a bit stronger and more flexible, have more energy, lose some weight (I can testify to this one), reduce stress and anxiety (and high blood pressure), improve concentration and memory, and feel more optimistic.

These are just a few of the general benefits of yoga practice. The specific benefits of each of the poses are noted in the text.

the ABCs of practice

I could rattle off a long list of elements of practice The most important elements are what I call the ABCs of yoga: A is for physical alignment, B is for breath, and C is for consciousness or self-awareness. These ABCs are first learned and cultivated in yoga practice, and then applied to everyday life.

A IS FOR ALIGNMENT

Alignment, explains *Merriam-Webster's Collegiate Dictionary*, 10th ed., is "the proper positioning or state of adjustment of parts . . . in relation to each other." The parts to be aligned, in the context of an asana practice, are parts of the body: the arms, legs, torso, neck, and head. Not all yoga schools are picky about physical alignment in asana, but my training insists that it's the foundation of the entire practice, the necessary precursor to psychological and spiritual alignment or, as the yogis say, equanimity (*samatva*). Much of what I've learned about alignment is based on the work of B. K. S. Iyengar, the yoga master who was born in 1918 and resides in Pune, India.

When you are in proper alignment, your body is anchored solidly to the Earth and at the same time you feel weightless and illuminated. Then the normally perceived limits of your body image expand, and you become psychologically spacious and pass naturally into a meditative frame of mind. To get a taste of what it feels like to be in alignment, try this exercise:

Exercise

1. Sit comfortably on the front edge of your chair seat, with your thighs

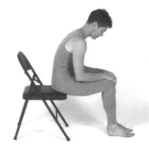
Alignment exercise: step 1

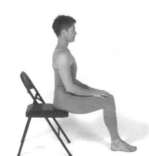
Alignment exercise: step 2

parallel and your knees at right angles. Rest your hands on your thighs. Close your eyes. Now slump your torso forward, exaggerating the rounding of your back and neck. *Stay here for a couple of minutes. How do you feel?*

2. Then, to the best of your ability, sit up "straight": make yourself as long as possible, and align your head lightly with the top of your spine (instead of letting it hang off the front side). *Again stay for a couple of minutes. How do you feel now? Any different?*

B IS FOR BREATH

The rules of breathing in yoga are straightforward: every time you fold your torso toward your leg or legs (such as when moving into a forward bend), or move your limb or limbs toward your torso (such as when lowering a raised arm to your side), you should exhale; every time you lift your torso away from your leg or legs (such as when moving out of a forward bend), or move a limb or limbs away from your torso, you should inhale.

When holding a pose, breathe through your nose (not your mouth), breathe as softly and smoothly as possible, and never hold your breath

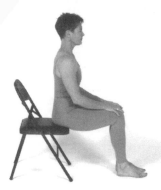

Breath exercise: step 1

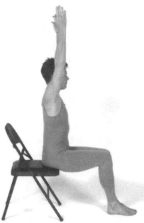

Breath exercise: step 2

(or at least be aware if you are holding your breath). Remember that there's an especially strong tendency to hold the breath in back bends (pages 98–111), but just about any pose you find challenging might cause you to stop breathing. If this happens, then either back off the pose slightly or come out of it completely: don't try to grimace and grunt your way through. Try this simple breathing exercise:

Exercise

1. Sit comfortably on the front edge of your chair seat, with your thighs parallel and your knees at right angles. Hang your arms by your sides.

2. Inhale and sweep your arms out to your sides and up. The arms should be parallel to each other and perpendicular to the floor. Hold for 10 to 15 seconds, breathing softly and smoothly through your nose. Then exhale and slowly lower your arms to your sides again. Wait a few breaths and repeat. Do this 4 or 5 times. *Be sure to keep your shoulders down, away from your ears.*

C IS FOR CONSCIOUSNESS

What is consciousness? The English word *conscious* is rooted in the Latin verb *scire*, "to know," which, in turn, is rooted in a word meaning "to cut." In order to be conscious, you need to "cut" your world into two pieces, a knowing subject—me—and a known object—everything and everyone else. In addition, you can also be conscious of your own body and the contents of your inner world. This means that the knower, which you usually imagine to be part and parcel of that inner world, is really somehow distinct from it; and moreover, the knower itself, no matter how hard you try to catch a glimpse of it, can't itself be known. Usually, unless you're a highly trained meditator, this knower is mostly submerged in and swept along by the inner world, and not all that aware of its own separate existence.

The yogis call the knower, which they often associate with the self, the "Witness" (*sakshin*). One goal of yoga is

to cultivate and refine the Witness, so that it can permanently rise above the constant stream of contents and remain fixedly detached from it. It's relatively easy to detach yourself from your inner world; the hard part is maintaining that distance for more than a few seconds. Try this exercise:

Exercise

1. Sit comfortably on the front edge of your chair seat, with your thighs parallel and your knees at right angles. Rest your hands on your thighs. Close your eyes.

2. Scan your body, starting with your feet and slowly moving up to your head. Take a couple of minutes to do this. Settle your awareness in (for example) your right hand, your left ear, or your belly—wherever you like. Recognize that although you inhabit this body, and love it dearly, some aspect of "you" can stand back from it and simply observe. Watch your thoughts, feelings, and sensations come and go. Don't judge them or try to influence them in any way: just watch as objectively as possible.

The observer in this exercise is the Witness, the unseen but all-seeing seer. What distinguishes yoga practice from other forms of exercise is the quality and quantity of your consciousness: the undivided and immediate presence of the Witness. Yoga done mechanically or unconsciously isn't really yoga: it's just exercise or gymnastics.

miscellaneous practice tips

TIME AND FREQUENCY

For a beginner, it's reasonable to set a short-term goal of thirty minutes, four times a week. It's natural to be zealous when you begin, but it's wiser to rein yourself in, start slowly, and gradually build up the amount of time you practice and the level of intensity.

Set aside a specific time when you know—and everyone who needs you knows—that you'll be busy with yoga. It's important to be regular if you want to see concrete results from your practice.

PLACE

Practice in a quiet place, as far away as possible from distractions, in an area that puts you in the mood to spend some quality time with yourself.

CLOTHING

A T-shirt and shorts is a fine yoga uniform, as is a leotard and tights. Bare feet are recommended, especially for the standing poses.

FOOD

Wait about an hour after eating a light snack to begin your practice, two hours if you've had a big, heavy meal.

ILLNESS AND INJURY

If you have a mild cold, a few of the gentler poses might help alleviate some of your misery. But if you're suffering the effects of a debilitating cold or flu, take some time off until you're feeling better.

Some injuries can be treated with the right kind of practice—and here I emphasize the word "right"—but others should be treated with rest. The best thing to do with an injury—to your knee, your back, or your neck, for example—is to consult an experienced teacher.

PAIN

You have to be able to distinguish between good pain—pain that says, *Ouch, this is really working*—and bad pain—pain that says, *Ouch, something's wrong here*. This will take some time and experience.

Inevitably, you're going to undergo some discomfort when you start your practice, in areas such as the backs of your legs or your shoulders. This is usually good pain, pain that will, with consistent practice, diminish and eventually transform itself into a pleasurable sensation.

Bad pain usually manifests in your joints, such as your knees, low back, or neck. Bad pain will, if you grit your teeth and soldier on, transform itself into an injury. At first, be conservative. Closely witness *any* pain, and be willing to back off for a while or even stop. Look carefully at the photos of the models in this book. Notice if your performance of the pain-inducing pose is somehow different from the model's, and make adjustments accordingly. If the pain persists, stop, and before you try the pose again, consult with an experienced teacher.

Stop exercising right away if you become dizzy or nauseous, experience pain in your upper body, break into a cold sweat, get pale, or (needless to say) faint.

props

Props are like training wheels on a kid's two-wheel bike. They help her make the transition from a tricycle to a two-wheeler, and give her the *feel* of doing something she ordinarily couldn't do. Of course, eventually the training wheels have to come off. Similarly, you'll eventually want to put aside your props—or at least depend on them less and less—as your practice develops.

The instruction in this book, influenced as it is by the Iyengar style of practice (which relies heavily on props in beginning classes), uses the following props:

STICKY MAT

A sticky mat is useful if your practice surface is carpeted or hard but slippery. If you're practicing on a bare wooden or tile floor, you may be able to work without a mat.

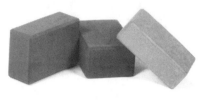

Foam blocks

BLOCK

Blocks are generally made of either wood or foam. Wooden blocks are heavy, and when used as a support they're very stable. Foam blocks are light, but they're less stable as supports.

If you don't want to invest in a block, you could use a piece of wood measuring about 3 x 5 x 8 (or 9) inches. Be sure to sand the block or wrap it in masking tape to protect yourself from splinters. A block has two ends, two sides, and two faces. The ends measure 3 x 5 inches. The sides 3 x 8 inches, and the faces 5 x 8 inches.

STRAP WITH BUCKLE

The best strap is made from cotton webbing and is at least five to six feet long. If you don't want to buy a strap, then use a strip of heavy cloth. When you need to tie yourself up with the strap, a buckle will come in handy, although you could just knot the strip of cloth.

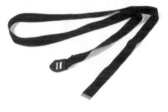

Strap with buckle

BLANKETS

Your blankets should be firm, made of wool or a wool/synthetic blend. One blanket is the minimum needed. It's better to have at least three blankets.

In this book, I'll use the following blanket terminology: fold a blanket in half, and look at the two sides; one side is "firm" (the side where the blanket has been folded), and one side is "open" (the side opposite the firm side). Whenever you sit or lie on a blanket (or blankets), be sure to use the firm side (or sides). This is especially important

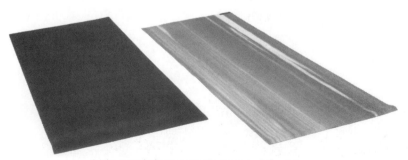

Sticky mats help prevent slipping on slick surfaces.

when using blankets to support your shoulders in All-Limb Pose (page 116), Plow (page 118), or Bridge (page 114).

FOLDING CHAIR
A common metal folding chair is a versatile yoga prop. If you don't want to buy one, you might be able to use a kitchen or dining room chair; just be sure it's *very* sturdy.

SAND BAG
Twenty or so years ago, the sand bag actually was filled with sand, but nowadays the bag is filled with some kind of plastic particles. It's used to weigh down parts like the thighs or shoulders in order to help release tension.

EYE BAG
An eye bag is a welcome prop for relaxation (page 128). The bag is usually made of silk, and filled with plastic pellets.

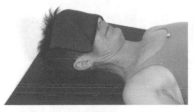

Eye bag

TIMER
It's a good idea to have a watch or clock handy when you practice. That way, with certain poses (such as Triangle Pose or Head-to-Knee Pose), you'll be sure to hold the two sides an equal length of time.

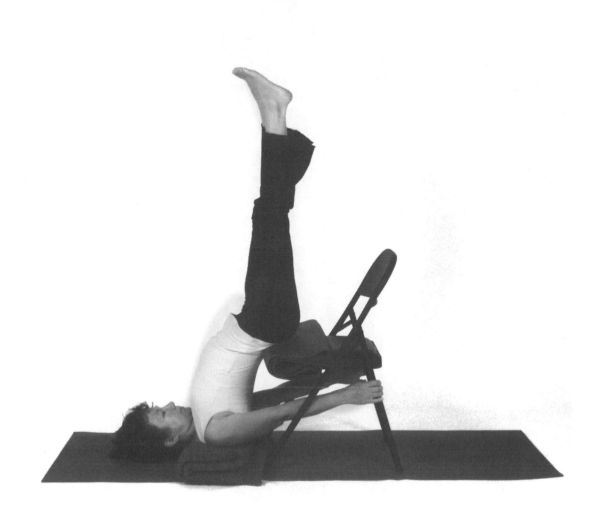

part two:

preliminary exercises

pieces of the puzzle

You've no doubt, at some time in your life, put together a jigsaw puzzle. When the pieces are rightly snapped in place you get a beautiful picture, but if you try to force pieces together that don't really fit, or leave out some pieces, then you get what my grandmother called a mishmash, and maybe even some broken pieces.

Think of the yoga asanas as jigsaw puzzles, each with its own pieces. Put these pieces together properly and you get a beautiful picture, with all the parts harmoniously aligned; but put the pieces together improperly, or try to leave some out, then you get another mishmash, and maybe even an injury.

Like regular puzzles, asana puzzles are different from one another; but unlike regular puzzles, asana puzzles have many pieces in common. The regular puzzle pieces are made of cardboard and thus static and fundamentally isolated from one another, even when one piece is plugged into its neighbor; asana-puzzle pieces are dynamic and interactive, no matter how far apart on the body they are. Every time

you adjust one piece, that adjustment ripples through all the other pieces like a wave.

Twelve exercises in Part II serve as preliminaries to the asanas in Part III. Each exercise reveals and establishes a different common piece of the puzzle, and in all but two (Exercises 1 and 10, Part II) you can see and/or touch concrete parts of the body—kneecaps, shoulder blades, ribs.

The instructions below involve either movements or actions (this terminology thanks to B. K. S. Iyengar). A movement is something you can do, like raise your arm in front of your torso. An action is something you can only imagine; for example, you can't "lengthen your tailbone," but you can *pretend* that you're doing it.

Actions involve imaginary lines or "channels" that, taken together, form an energetic network that criss-cross the body, both on its surface and through its interior. When visualized in this way, our body image is fluid, more open to change, and less monolithic. You can use these channels as a:

- Preparation for your upcoming practice while lying in Corpse (page 128).
- Framework to direct (or harness) the flow of energy during asana or pranayama practice.
- Focus during relaxation at the end of practice, again lying in Corpse.

The channels feed and/or support the "core" of the body, or the "front" spine, which we'll learn more about in the exercises below, especially in Exercise 10.

Be sure to read through this section before you try the exercises, and then be sure to practice the exercises before you continue on to Part III. Don't hurry to get through the exercises. They're important! Take time to understand each one before you move to the next. The descriptions of these exercises won't be repeated in the instructions for the asanas. It'll be up to you to remember to fit them properly into the asana-puzzle you're working on.

PROPS: A sticky mat, a block (preferably foam), and a wall.

EXERCISE 1: THE HEADS OF THE THIGHBONES

The ball-shaped heads of the thighbones (femur) nestle in the hip sockets, to either side of the pubis. For most people, the femur heads are misaligned in their sockets, so energy that should be freely flowing to the heels and spine is stuck in the pelvis.

PRELIMINARY PRACTICE: WHERE ARE THE FEMUR HEADS?

1. Lie on your back, knees bent, feet on the floor, heels about 12 inches away from your buttocks, inner thighs parallel. Exhale and lift your right foot away from the floor.

2. Slowly circle your thigh clockwise, drawing a large circle on the ceiling with your kneecap. Gradually make the circle increasingly smaller until the movement stops.

3. When you stop circling, see if you can feel how the femur head sinks into the hip socket. Circle the right leg counterclockwise for approximately the same number of turns, then repeat both circles with your left leg.

MAIN PRACTICE

1. Stand with your back to a wall, heels 12 inches off the wall, inner feet parallel. Wedge the sides of the block between your top back thighs and the wall. Your buttocks should be *above* the block, as if sitting on its top face.

2. Exhale and bend forward until your torso is about parallel to the floor. Careful! Don't drop the block. Push your hands to the wall at hip height, and press your top thighs firmly against the block.

3. After holding this position for 30 seconds, exhale and lower into a forward bend. Continue to press your thighs actively against the block. From the action of the femur heads, burrow your heels into the floor and lengthen your front torso away from your groins. Continue for 2 to 3 minutes.

Benefit

This exercise centers the pelvis on the heads of the femurs, which grounds the heels and lengthens the spine.

Caution

If you tend to lock your knees (rather than press your thighs), see Exercise 4.

Tip

If you tip forward as you lean into the forward bend, move your feet a few inches farther from the wall.

EXERCISE 2: THE FEET AND ANKLES

Remove the block and rest your buttocks against the wall. If you can't easily touch your feet with your knees straight, bend your knees as much as you need to.

MAIN PRACTICE

1. With your thumbs, press the mounds of your big toes (but not your big toes themselves) firmly against the floor. Stroke your thumbs back along the inner arches from the mounds to the inner heels several times. As you

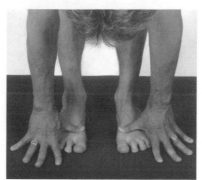

Press firmly on the mounds of the big toes, not the big toes themselves.

continue to press the mounds, stroke your fingers along the outer edges of the feet from the heels to the little toes, then imagine your little toes growing out onto the floor.

2. Hook your thumbs under your inner ankles and your fingers under your outer ankles. Pinch the bones together by narrowing the space between each pair of bones; simultaneously widen the heels.

3. Pull your inner ankles up, as if lifting them toward your inner groins, then stroke up your inner legs. Repeat several times. Imagine drawing energy from the earth along your inner legs and up through your groins and deep into your pelvis.

Benefit

The actions of the feet and ankles center the weight of the body on the ankle joints and lessen the tendency to collapse onto the inner arch.

Tip

If you have difficulty experiencing the lift of the inner arches, lift your toes away from the floor and watch how this movement strengthens the inner arches. Then soften the toes back onto the floor, but maintain the lift of the arches.

EXERCISE 3: THE INNER GROINS

The groins are located where the thighs join the pelvis.

PRELIMINARY PRACTICE: WHERE ARE THE INNER GROINS?

With your buttocks on the wall, bend your knees slightly. Slide your fingertips into the creases between your inner thighs and the bottom of your pelvis (perineum). Gently trace the course of these creases from either side of the pubis to their respective sitting bones and back again a few times. These are the inner groins.

Then push your hands against the wall and swing into a full standing forward bend, straightening your knees, legs more or less perpendicular to the floor.

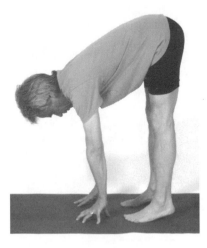

Main Practice: Inner Groins
Don't lift your heels too high; only an inch or so is enough.

MAIN PRACTICE

1. Rest your fingertips on the floor (or a block if the floor is too far away), lean forward onto the balls of your feet, and raise your heels an inch away from the floor. Imagine drawing your inner groins up into your pelvis, as if lifting them toward your sacrum. You might be able to feel also how, when you do this, the perineum domes up slightly.

2. Without losing the lift of the inner groins, slowly return your heels to the floor. Descend your outer heels faster than the inner. Your inner legs should feel slightly longer than your outer legs.

Benefit

This action further balances the pelvis and lengthens the spine.

Tip

If you want to take this exercise a little further, think not only of lifting the inner groins, but widening them as well. After lifting, imagine them spreading toward your outer hips.

EXERCISE 4: THE KNEES

Here are two exercises for the knees: one for people with "straight" knees, the other for people with "locked" knees. With straight knees, the kneecaps will face forward, and a line drawn down the middle of your outer leg from the hip to the ankle will pass through the middle of your outer knee. With locked knees, the kneecaps will turn slightly inward, and that outer-leg line will pass slightly in *front* of the middle knee. Locked knees block the

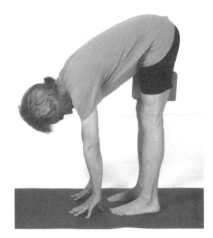

Main Practice: Straight Knees
Squeeze the block firmly, but be sure not to harden your inner groins and the backs of your knees.

downward flow of energy to the feet, and risk injury.

Slide your block between your thighs, a few inches above your knees, sides touching your inner thighs.

MAIN PRACTICE: STRAIGHT KNEES

1. Squeeze the block with your front thigh muscles (quadriceps); as you do, your kneecaps will lift. Contract and release your quadriceps several times to feel the movement of your kneecaps.

2. Lift the kneecaps *up*, don't push them *back* into the joint. When you straighten the knees, don't harden the backs of the knees.

MAIN PRACTICE: LOCKED KNEES

1. Remove the block then bend forward. Notice your knees are slightly cross-eyed and pushed back. Bend them slightly and, with the bases of your palms, rotate your kneecaps outward until they face forward.

2. Press your hands against your calves. Contract your thighs and

lift your kneecaps. If you're used to locking your knees, straight knees will feel slightly bent. Whenever you perform any pose that requires straight knees, remember how this exercise feels and re-create the movements.

Benefit

This action strengthens the thighs and aligns the knees.

Tip

If you can't yet feel the lift of your kneecaps, cup your hands over them and "scrub" them up the front thighs, sliding your hands toward the groins.

EXERCISE 5. THE THIGHS

Thighs can rotate inward and outward. In some poses (e.g.,

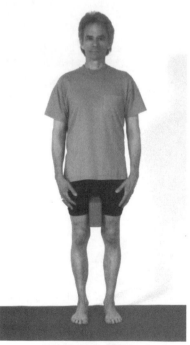

Main Practice: Thighs
You can press your hands lightly against your outer thighs. Press your outer thighs against the block as you widen your inner groins.

all the back bends) you want the former, while in others (e.g., Triangle Pose) the latter.

Inhale and, with the block still squeezed between your thighs, and with a long front torso, lift slowly to upright.

MAIN PRACTICE

1. While you're using your *inner* thigh muscles (adductors) to squeeze the block, pretend you're squeezing the block with your *outer* thigh muscles (abductors). When you firm the outer thighs, notice how your inner feet press more actively against the floor.

2. Slowly roll your thighs outward and push the block forward, then roll your thighs inward and push the block backward. Repeat several times, rotating your thighs through their full range of movement. Gradually come to a stop in what you feel is a neutral position between the two extremes, kneecaps looking straight forward.

Benefit

This exercise helps to center the femur heads in the hip sockets and balance the pelvis and spine.

Caution

Any time you strengthen your legs (as in the standing poses or Shoulder Stand), be sure not to harden your belly, groins, or outer hips.

Tip

In Part III, the following poses need inward rotation of the

legs: Intense Stretch and Powerful Pose; the three belly exercises; the two arm-strength poses; Staff, Hero, Reclining Big Toe, Head-to-Knee (straight leg only), Intense Stretch-of-the-West Poses; Marichi's Pose; the five back bends; and the inversions. For the rest of the poses, rotate the legs outward.

EXERCISE 6. THE SACRUM, HIP POINTS, AND TAILBONE

Sacrum literally means "sacred bone."

PRELIMINARY PRACTICE: WHERE ARE THE HIP POINTS?

Slide your index fingertips away and down slightly from your belly button, each for about 6 inches, until you find the pair of bony knobs (the hip points) that marks the top rim of your front pelvis.

MAIN PRACTICE

1. Resume rolling the block. Outward rotation widens your hip points, narrows your sacrum, "flattens" your front groins, and lengthens your tail down and presses it forward toward your pubis.

2. Roll the block back inward: your hip points narrow while your sacrum widens, your front groins "hollow," and your tail duck-tails out behind.

3. Roll the block forward and back several times, exaggerating these movements. Finally roll the block inward; without losing the narrowness of your hips, the width

of your sacrum, or the depth of your front groins, lengthen your tail down and press it slightly forward, as if you were (but aren't actually) rolling the block forward. If needed, use your hands to create the described movements/actions.

4. Stay for a minute or two.

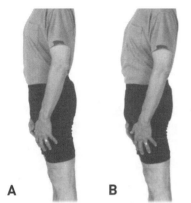

A   **B**

Be sure your pelvis doesn't tip forward (figure A); bring the top rim parallel to the floor (figure B).

Benefits

The wide sacrum softens the buttocks, increases the flexibility of the hips, and balances the pelvis on the femur heads. The narrow hip points engages the inner thigh muscles and psoas pair (page 58); also, with the wide sacrum, the narrow hips help balance the pelvis on the femur heads. These combined actions of the pelvis encourage the length of the spine.

Tip

Don't lengthen your tail by tucking it forward into the pelvis, which flattens the curve of your lower back. *Lengthen* your tail downward and "sharpen" it inward, but

always maintain the natural curves of your spine.

EXERCISE 7. THE ARMS

Like your legs, your arms can rotate either inward or outward. In most poses, you'll want to rotate your arms outward, though there are a few poses (e.g., Intense Stretch-of-the-East) that need inward rotation.

MAIN PRACTICE (1): ROTATING THE ARMS

1. Stand with your arms hanging alongside your torso. Turn your arms outward so your palms face forward and thumbs point out. Then turn your palms back, thumbs pointing in toward your torso. Rotate out and in several times with exaggerated movements. Notice how outward rotation opens your chest and squeezes your scapulae, inward rotation opens your back torso and collapses your chest.

2. Stretch your arms out to your sides, parallel to the floor. Outwardly rotate your arms, turning your palms up and releasing your scapulae down your back. Then inwardly rotate them, turning the palms down and lifting your scapulae toward your ears.

3. Raise your arms perpendicular to the floor but parallel to each other, palms facing in. Again rotate out and in. The former widens your back torso, the latter lifts your scapulae toward your ears.

Benefit

These actions help to center the humerus heads in the

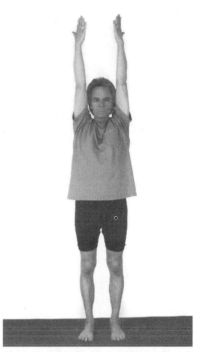

Keep the tops of your shoulders soft, and your shoulder blades releasing down your back.

shoulder sockets and balance the shoulder yoke on the torso.

Tip

In Part III, the following poses need inward rotation of the arms: Staff and Cow Face (initially for the lower arm, when bringing it into the first position); Locust and Intense-Stretch-of-the-East; Child's Pose (when the arms are beside the torso). In the rest of the poses, turn the arms outward.

EXERCISE 8: THE SHOULDER BLADES AND STERNUM

The top of the breastbone or sternum is called the manubrium, which means "handle," while the bottom tip is the xiphoid (pronounced ZIF-oid), which means "sword." The old anatomists who named this bone pictured it as a sword or knife, with its tip pointing down toward your navel and its handle just under the hollow at the front throat.

PROP: *You'll need a blanket roll about 6 to 8 inches in diameter.*

MAIN PRACTICE

1. Lie on the roll with lower scapulae supported, knees bent, feet on the floor. If the roll is positioned properly, your arms will rest comfortably on the floor out to your sides.

2. Reach your arms toward the ceiling, perpendicular to the floor and parallel to each other. Rock gently side to side and widen your scapulae across your back. Then, without losing that width, lay your arms on the floor.

3. Rest a fingertip on your manubrium. Imagine the roll is pressing your lower scapulae up and forward through your torso toward this point. Soften your upper chest to receive this action. Push your feet lightly against the floor to scrub the scapulae down your back.

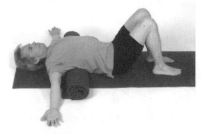

Your arms should rest comfortably on the floor. Continue to lengthen your tail toward your heels.

Benefit

The action of the scapulae helps lift the manubrium, which in turn balances the head atop the spine, releasing tension in the shoulders and neck and lengthening the front spine.

Tip

There's a tendency, when instructed to "lift your chest," to push your xiphoid forward, compressing your lower back, sharpening your front ribs, and hardening your belly. Instead, bring the xiphoid slightly down (toward your navel) and into your torso, and lift only your manubrium.

EXERCISE 9: THE RIBS

Each of the 12 pairs of ribs is rooted in a thoracic vertebra. The top seven pairs, the "true" ribs, are attached directly to the sternum. The five pairs of "false" ribs are attached only indirectly to the sternum or not at all (pairs 11 and 12, the "floating" ribs).

MAIN PRACTICE

1. Lie flat on the floor, knees bent, feet on the floor. Cross your arms over your chest and hold the heads of your upper arm bones (humerus) with the opposite-side hands.

2. Rock gently side to side. Pull your humerus heads together in front, and broaden your back ribs away from your spine. Then slip your hands down into the opposite-side

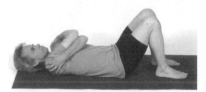

Hug yourself and widen your shoulder blades, but don't narrow your upper chest.

armpits and squeeze your side ribs. Imagine the side ribs slightly narrowing from armpit to armpit.

3. Slide your hands toward your sternum. Gently press the ribs into the sternum, and widen this bone against their resistance.

Benefits

Narrowing the ribcase helps release tension in the muscles between the ribs (intercostals) and those attached to the shoulder yoke, which in turn helps improve breathing. It also encourages the lift of the top sternum.

Tip

Also widen and lift your collar bones (clavicles). Rest your index fingertips on your top sternum, then slide them apart along the clavicles to the top of each shoulder (acromion). Repeat a few times. Then spread your fingertips under the clavicles and press them up, as if you were trying the push them over the tops of your shoulders. Feed this action into your shoulder blades as they slide down your back torso.

EXERCISE 10: THE FRONT AND BACK OF THE SPINE

In part 2 of this exercise, we'll search for the imaginary (or energetic) front spine, which runs straight from the middle of the perineum to the crown of the head. Don't despair if you can't find it immediately. Be patient and keep searching—it's worth the effort.

For this exercise, remain on your back with your knees bent.

MAIN PRACTICE (1): THE PHYSICAL BACK SPINE

1. Cross your arms over your chest and hold the heads of your humerus bones with the opposite-side hands.

2. Push your feet lightly against the floor. Imagine you're sliding along the floor in the direction of your head. Feel your physical back spine scrubbed downward from the inion (see Exercise 11) to your tail.

Tip

Be sure the inion (see Exercise 11) isn't dragged down onto the back of your neck. Lift it toward your crown, away from your descending back spine, to lengthen your nape.

MAIN PRACTICE (2): THE IMAGINARY FRONT SPINE

1. Pretend your torso is shaped like a cylinder (it's not). With your arms crossed, slowly rock from side to side on the curved surface of your torso-cylinder.

2. The axis of this rocking movement is an imaginary line passing through the center of your cylinder-torso. Continue gently rocking until you get a feel for this line. Then slowly stop your rocking and lie quietly on the floor, tracing your "front spine" in your imagination.

Benefit

The complementary actions of the spine provide a focus and organizing principle for all other actions and movements. These two channels embody the dual essence of our human nature: the urges to incarnate and to transcend.

Tip

Here's a mantra that will help you remember the actions of the spine in all your activities: "Up the front, down the back" (thanks to Mabel Todd).

EXERCISE 11. THE BASE OF THE SKULL AND THE CROOK OF THE THROAT

Most people squeeze the base of the skull, which pushes their chin forward and shortens the back of their neck (nape).

PRELIMINARY PRACTICE: WHERE IS THE BASE OF THE SKULL AND THE CROOK OF THE THROAT?

Find the bony knob at the back of your head, just where the nape meets the skull. This is the inion (or occipital protuberance), which marks what we're calling the base of the skull.

Find the bump of your larynx on the front of your throat. Just above this, where the underside of the chin meets the front throat, is a smile-shaped crease, which we're calling the crook of the throat.

Stay on your back with your knees bent.

MAIN PRACTICE

1. Hook your thumbs underneath inion and lift it away from the nape. Imagine that the inion is sliding away from the nape, opening a space between the two.

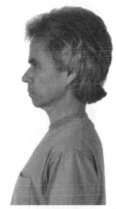

When your head is in balance over your spine, the head itself feels light and the back of the neck is relatively soft.

2. Notice how this action energetically tugs on the crook of your throat. Touch your index fingertips to your throat crook, to either side of your larynx, and *gently* press diagonally up and in.

Benefits

The actions of the inion and throat crook help lift the manubrium, and center your head on the top of the spine. They also help soften your throat and spread your tongue on the floor of your mouth.

Tip

How can you tell when your head is neutral? Looking from the side, your ear hole will be aligned over the center of your shoulder joint; from the front, your ears will be equidistant from your shoulders, and the tip of your nose over the middle of your sternum.

EXERCISE 12: PUTTING IT ALL TOGETHER

When practicing the yoga asanas in this book, you'll want to automatically apply what you've learned in all the exercises, except the two limb rotation exercises (5 and 7), which are situational.

For this exercise we'll work on two representative yoga asanas: *Mountain Pose*, the basic standing pose, and *Downward Facing Dog Pose*.

MOUNTAIN POSE

Tadasana (tah-DAHS-anna)
tada = mountain

Mountain is every asana's foundation, but especially the standing poses. Just as there's a mythic mountain, Mount Meru, at the center of Hinduism's universe, so is there a mountain at the center of our practice, representing a "bridge" between our mundane world and the divine.

1. Stand with your inner feet parallel and a few inches apart, thighs rotated slightly inward. Lift and spread the balls of your feet, then release them back to the floor.

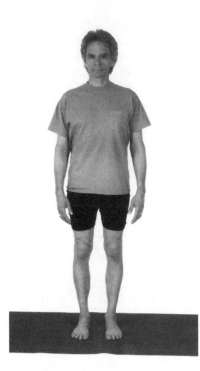

Mountain Pose

2. Excluding Exercises 5 and 7, run through and apply what you learned in the previous exercises. Hang your arms alongside your torso, palms facing your hips. Gaze straight ahead. Stay for 1 to 3 minutes.

Benefit

Mountain strengthens your thighs, knees, and ankles, and improves posture.

Tip

To check your alignment in Mountain, perform the pose against a wall. Stand with your heels a couple of inches from the wall, and rest your buttocks and shoulder blades (but not the back of your head) against the wall.

DOWNWARD FACING DOG POSE

Adho Mukha Shvanasana (ah-doh moo-kah shvah-NAHS-anna)

adho mukha = face downward (adho = downward; mukha = face); shvana = dog

Many yoga poses are named after living creatures, and it's reasonable to speculate the yogis "invented" these poses by mimicking their namesakes. Downward Facing Dog is one of the simplest but most useful of the asanas.

1. Get down on your hands and knees, hands slightly forward of your shoulders, knees directly below your hips. Spread your palms and fingers broadly, and adjust your index fingers in one of two ways: if you're tighter in your shoulders, turn them out

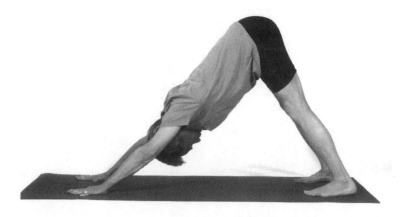

Downward Facing Dog Pose

slightly; if your shoulders are open, set them parallel to each other.

2. Rotate your upper arms outward. Your elbow creases will turn forward and the weight on your hands will shift onto the pinky sides. Without losing that rotation, press the bases of your index fingers firmly into the floor.

3. Turn your toes under, exhale, lift your knees away from the floor, and straighten your knees. Review your exercise lessons. Turn your thighs slightly inward and align your ears between your upper arms. Stretch your heels toward the floor, outer heels descending faster than the inner. Stay for 1 to 3 minutes, then release your knees with an exhale to the floor.

Benefit
Downward Facing Dog strengthens the arms and legs, and stretches the shoulders and chest, hamstrings, and calves. It's a "neutralizing" pose, calming you when you're stressed, and invigorating you when you're tired.

Caution
Avoid this pose with high blood pressure.

Tip
If your neck feels strained in this pose, support your forehead on one end of a block positioned between your upper arms.

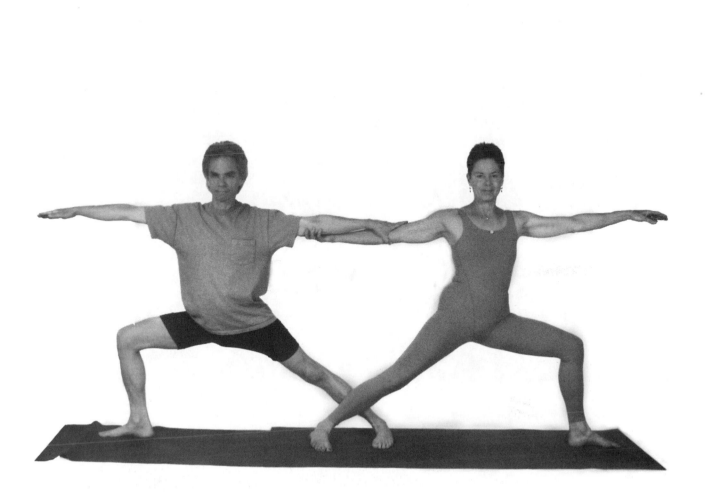

part three:

the poses

ent-Knee Lunge

ent-Knee Lunge is a preparation for most poses and the Sun Salute (see page 30).

Perform with the right leg then repeat with the left

1 Kneel on a folded blanket in the middle of your sticky mat. Step your right foot forward to the right front corner of the mat. Slide your left knee back until you feel a comfortable stretch across the front thigh and groin. *Note: Turn your right foot slightly out to the right.*

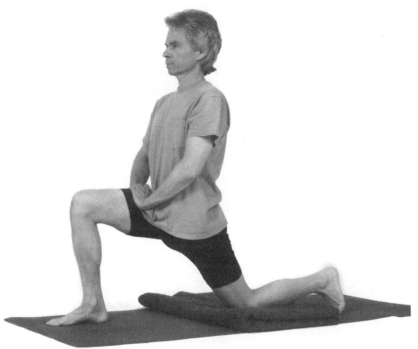

BENEFITS

Opens the groin and softens the inner groin of the front (bent-knee) leg, and stretches the front groin and the psoas of the back (straight) leg.

TIPS

You can hold this lunge static and just let your torso be drawn downward by gravity, or you can swing your torso away from, or twist it toward, the bent knee.

2 Lean your torso forward and rest your hands on the floor. Slide your back knee as much as you can away from your pelvis. Hold for 1 to 2 minutes. *Note: Press your right shoulder against the inside of your right thigh. Rotate your right thigh out, roll your right hip in. Be sure to keep your front knee over the ankle.*

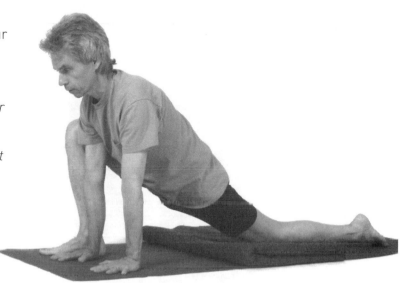

3 If flexibility permits, lay your forearms on the floor. *Note: Be sure to keep your front knee over the ankle.*

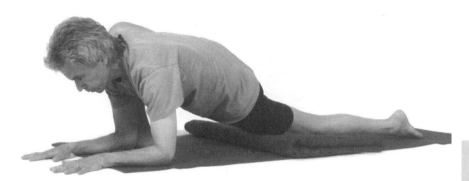

To Come Up: Inhale your torso up and step your front knee back beside your back knee.

Sun Salute

Surya Namaskar (soor-yah nah-MAHS-car)
surya = Sun; namaskar = to salute, pay homage to

Sun Salute is an excellent warm-up for an asana practice, or it can be used as a mini-practice in itself on those days when time is short. There are many variations of Sun Salute. The sequence we'll work with consists of 13 "stations" composed of eight different poses, the last five being the same as the first five, except performed in reverse order.

The sequence begins and ends in Mountain. Each movement is coordinated with either an inhale or an exhale. Be sure to stay conscious of your breath as you move through the sequence. Slow down if your breathing struggles, take a short rest if your breathing stops altogether. As you do for the asanas, always breathe through your nose, never your mouth.

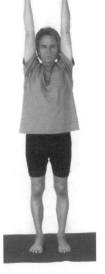

1 MOUNTAIN POSE (page 24): Stand with your inner feet parallel. Hang your arms alongside your torso, palms facing your hips.

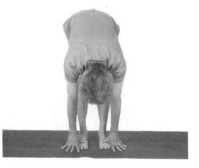

2 RAISED-ARMS MOUNTAIN POSE (Urdhva Hasta Tadasana): Inhale, sweep your arms out to your sides, and stretch them upward. Fix your arms parallel to each other and extend a little more through the pinky-sides of your hands. If it doesn't strain your neck or shoulders, press your palms together above your head.

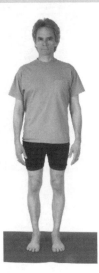

3 STANDING FORWARD BEND (page 52): Exhale, sweep your arms out to your sides, and fold forward and down. Press your fingertips on the floor.

The sequence shown (steps 1–13) completes one *half-round*. Repeat, substituting "left" for "right" and "right" for "left" where appropriate. Now that's one round. Start your practice with maybe 3 rounds and gradually work your way up to 10 to 15. If you like to sweat, go as fast as you reasonably can, but if you want a more contemplative practice, slow your pace down. In either case, move consciously, especially as you near the end of your practice, when weariness often leads to sloppiness. Remember that, like all the asanas, Sun Salute only improves with regular practice.

4 LUNGE: Inhale and step your left foot back into a lunge. Position your right knee directly over your right ankle, and press actively through your left heel. If you find it difficult to keep your left leg long and straight, bend that knee to the floor.

5 DOWNWARD FACING DOG (page 24): Exhale and step your right foot back to Downward Facing Dog.

6 PLANK: Inhale and swing your torso forward into Plank. Position your shoulders over your wrists, firm your thighs, and lengthen your tail; be sure your lower back doesn't sag.

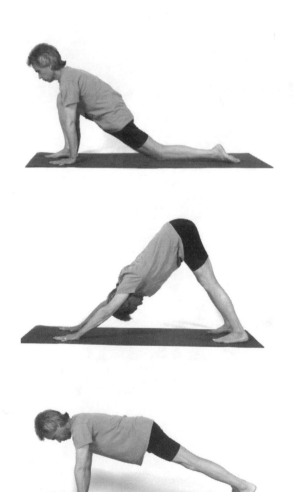

Sun Salute *continued*

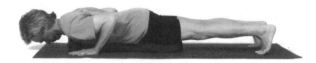

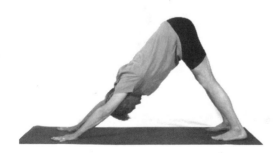

7 FOUR-LIMB STAFF POSE (page 68): Exhale and lower to Four-Limb Staff.

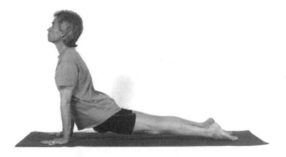

8 UPWARD FACING DOG (page 110): Inhale and sweep your torso to Upward Facing Dog.

9 DOWNWARD FACING DOG: Exhale back to Downward Facing Dog, generating the movement by pressing your femur bones actively away from the floor.

10 LUNGE: Inhale and step your right foot back to Lunge. If you find this difficult or impossible, bend your knees to the floor, step the foot back between the hands, then raise the bent knee again.

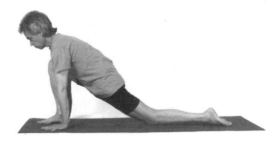

BENEFITS

One obvious benefit of the Sun Salute is that just about anyone can do it. It's also claimed to:

- Improve strength, flexibility, and endurance.
- Help slim the belly, hips, and thighs, improve posture and balance, and promote graceful movement.

- Increase the strength and efficiency of the heart, and improve blood circulation.
- Ventilate the lungs of toxic gases and increase lung capacity.
- Tone and massage the belly organs (like the liver, stomach, and intestines).
- Relieve tension, calm the brain, and develop concentration.

CAUTIONS

Avoid Sun Salute if you have high blood pressure, a herniated spinal disk, sciatica, or an inguinal hernia.

11 STANDING FORWARD BEND: Exhale your left foot back to Standing Forward Bend. Keep the leg straight and active as you swing it forward.

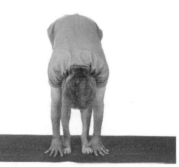

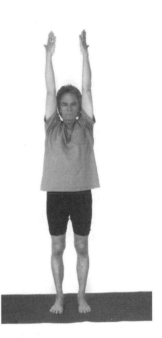

12 RAISED-ARMS MOUNTAIN POSE: Inhale and sweep your arms to the sides and up for Raised-Arms Mountain.

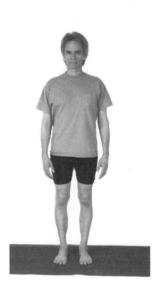

13 MOUNTAIN POSE: Exhale your hands back together and return your arms down alongside your torso.

standing poses

The standing poses in this section are the foundation of the entire asana practice. Your early practice of asana should rely heavily on the standing poses, which generally strengthen the legs, ankles, and spine; open the groins; and build a sense of balance (both physical and emotional) and self-confidence.

There are two kinds of standing poses: one-sided, with your feet aligned and parallel; and two-sided, with your feet unaligned and at different angles.

TIPS

Generally, in the one-sided poses, your feet should be parallel to each other and a few inches apart, your heels below your hips. This slight opening broadens your base of support and makes you more stable; however, if you want to challenge your balance, narrow your base of support by touching the bases of your big toes and separating your heels about an inch.

In the two-sided poses, beginning students with shorter legs should allow maybe 3 to 3½ feet between their feet; those with longer legs should allow 3½ to 4 feet. Be aware,

though, that some of the more challenging standing poses (Revolved Triangle, Warrior 1, and Intense Side Stretch poses) are slightly easier to perform with the feet closer together.

Additionally, in the two-sided standing poses, roll the back-leg hip slightly forward so that hip is a bit closer to the edge of the mat than its front-leg mate.

In the two-sided poses, your front foot is always turned out 90 degrees; in other words, as you're facing the long edge of your mat with your feet parallel, pivot on your front-foot heel and turn the foot from 12 o'clock to 3 o'clock. Your back foot always turns in (toward the front foot), but less with some poses and more with others. For most poses, pivot your back foot toward the front-foot side about 30 degrees; in a few of the poses, though (Revolved Triangle, Virabhadra 1, and Intense Side Stretch poses), turn your back foot in about 60 degrees.

In three of the standing poses (Extended Side Angle, and Virabhadra I and II poses), your front knee bends: if you're more flexible in the

groins, you'll bend until your shin is perpendicular and your thigh is parallel to the floor (so your knee is in a right angle); if you're less flexible, bring your shin perpendicular to the floor, but don't worry if your thigh is slightly above parallel (so that your knee is angled at more than 90 degrees).

There are two recommended foot alignments for the two-sided poses. Usually, the heel of your front foot is in line with the midarch of your back foot, but many beginners find this alignment somewhat unstable. You also align your front heel with your back heel to provide a broader base of support.

Stand in the middle of your sticky mat, facing one of its long edges (it's traditional when practicing yoga to face either to the East or North, which are considered to be the "propitious" quarters of the compass). All standing poses in this section begin and end in Mountain Pose (see page 24). You can either spring your feet lightly apart, or (if you have any injuries to your ankles or spine) simply step your feet apart to the recommended distance.

CAUTIONS

It's especially important to remember the knee–ankle alignment discussed in Part II (see page 19) when performing the two-sided poses. As you ready yourself for the pose, always rotate your front thigh outward so that the "eye" of your kneecap is looking out over (is in line with) the middle of the same-side ankle (the point midway between the two anklebones). This rotation will tend to shift your weight onto the outside edge of your front foot; to counter this, press actively through the base of your big toe and inner heel.

In the three bent-knee poses, it's essential that you keep your front knee aligned with your front ankle. When bending your knee (on an exhalation), aim the inner knee toward the little-toe side of your foot; don't "circle" your knee first inward and then back out over your ankle.

Another caution applies to several of the two-sided poses (Triangle, Revolved Triangle, Extended Side Angle, Virabhadra II, and Half Moon poses). Many popular instructional manuals show the practitioner's head turned toward the top, or front, arm. But this is not always appropriate for beginners. In order to safely turn your head, you first have to be able to lengthen your neck and align your head in a neutral position. So at the beginning, gaze forward at the opposite wall. This caution especially applies if you have any neck injury.

PROPS

Two props are indispensable for beginning students when practicing the standing poses. The first is a block. In many of the standing poses (for example, Triangle Pose), one hand (the "bottom" hand in the pose) is pressed against the floor. Beginners frequently have a difficult time comfortably touching the floor with the hand, or even with the fingertips. Use your block to support the hand, preferably with the palm flat (not the fingertips) on either one end, the side, or the face.

The second prop is a wall. Many beginners are unsteady in the standing poses. There are two ways to use the wall: either practice with your entire backside against the wall, or with your back-leg heel anchored in the corner between the wall and floor.

Tree Pose

Vrkshasana (vriks-SHAHS-anna)

vrksha = tree

Perform with the left leg then repeat with the right

"Look after the root of the tree and the fragrant flowers and luscious fruits will grow by themselves. Look after the health of the body, and the fragrance of the mind and richness of the spirit will flow" (from B. K. S. Iyengar, *Iyengar: His Life and Work*, 536).

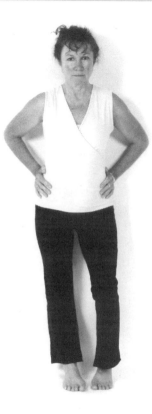

1 Stand with your heels a few inches from a wall, then lean your back against it. Inhale and shift your weight onto your right leg. *Note: Press the inside of your right foot firmly to the floor and align your spine directly over your right foot.*

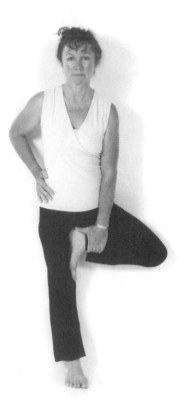

2 Exhale, raise your left foot, grasp the ankle, and place the sole against your inner right thigh. *Note: Point your toes toward the floor and spread the raised sole against your thigh.*

BENEFITS

Strengthens the thighs and ankles; stretches the groins, inner thighs, and chest; and improves your sense of balance.

CAUTION

When bringing the bent-knee foot up in this pose, there's a tendency for the standing foot to turn out, which could strain the standing-leg knee. Be sure to keep the standing foot pointing straight forward.

CHALLENGE YOURSELF

Tree Pose is normally a free-standing balance pose. To increase the challenge in this pose, perform it away from the wall. Also, try to tuck the raised heel into the standing-leg groin.

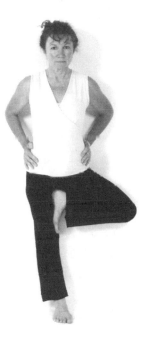

3 Firming the outer right thigh against the pressure of your left foot, release your ankle and rest your hands on your hips. *Note: Make sure your pelvis is neutral, its rim parallel to the floor and the two hip points equidistant from the wall opposite. Don't push your left knee back; hold it slightly forward of the right leg.*

4 Press your palms together and rest your thumbs on your sternum. Fix your gaze on a point on the floor about 4 or 5 feet away. Stay for 30 seconds to 1 minute.

To Come Up: Step the raised foot back to Mountain with an exhale.

Triangle Pose

Trikonasana (trik-cone-AHS-anna)
tri = three; kona = angle (trikona = triangle)

Many poses take their names from the way they look. There are actually three triangles formed in this pose: one triangle formed by the legs and floor, another by the bottom arm, front leg, and underside of the torso, and a third triangle with the hand, floor, and back of the front heel.

1 Spread your feet 3 to 4 feet apart. Turn your right foot out 90 degrees, your left foot in about 30 degrees. Set a block on one end outside your right foot. Rest your hands on your hips. *Note: Make sure your left heel is actively pressed to the floor (or against the corner of the room) to anchor the pose.*

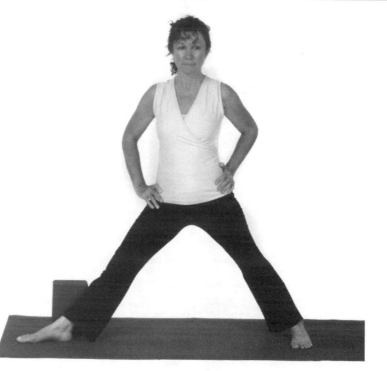

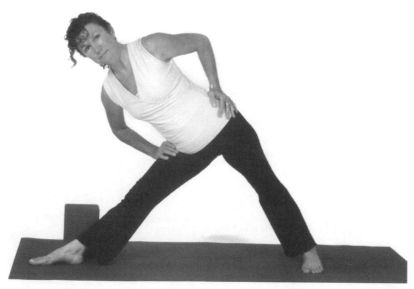

2 Exhale, shift your pelvis to the left and tip your torso to the right, over the plane of your right leg. *Note: Make sure to draw your right groin deep into your pelvis as you tip down. Depending on your flexibility, stop when your spine is more or less parallel to the floor.*

BENEFITS

Stretches and strengthens the thighs, knees, and ankles; stretches the groins, hamstrings, calves, and shoulders.

TIP

Make sure to lengthen the underside of your torso and don't hump the top side up toward the ceiling.

CHALLENGE YOURSELF

In time, you should be able to do away with the block and be able to bring your hand flat to the floor.

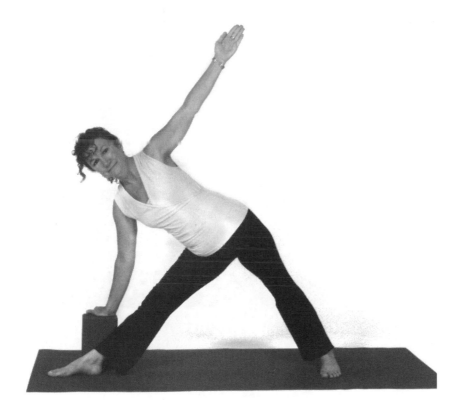

3 Turn your upper torso to the left. Reach down and press your right palm against the end of the block, then inhale and extend your left arm toward the ceiling. Hold for 30 seconds to 1 minute. *Note: Don't push your left hip back. Roll it slightly forward and rotate your rib case to the right. Stretch your tail toward your left heel to lengthen your lower back.*

To Come Up: Inhale and actively press down through your back heel as you reach up through your raised arm.

Revolved Triangle Pose

Parivrtta trikonasana (par-ee-vrit-tah trik-cone-AHS-anna)
parivrtta = to turn around, revolve; trikona = three angle or triangle

Several of the standing poses have revolved or twisted variations. Revolved Triangle (the only one included in this book) is, of course, a twisted variation of the previous pose, Triangle.

1 Spread your feet 3 to 4 feet apart. Turn your right foot out 90 degrees, your left foot in about 60 degrees. Set your yoga block inside your right foot. Rest your hands on your hips. *Note: Make sure your heels are aligned and your left heel is actively pressed to the floor (or against the corner of the room) to anchor the pose.*

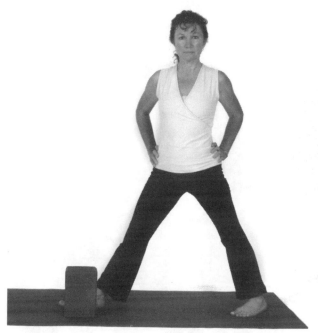

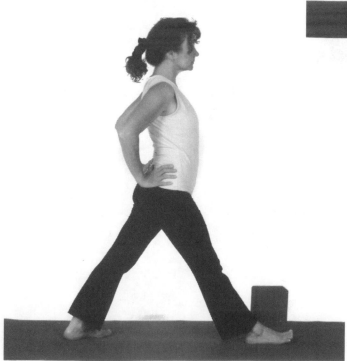

2 With an exhale, turn your torso to the right as close to 90 degrees as is comfortable while keeping your left leg straight.

BENEFITS

Strengthens and stretches the legs; and stretches the outer hips, chest, and spine.

CAUTIONS

Avoid this pose if you have any serious spine or neck injury.

TIP

If you have difficulty keeping the back heel grounded, raise it on a support, such as a sand bag or thickly folded mat.

3 Inhale, lift your chest, then exhale and lower your torso as close to parallel to the floor as is comfortable. *Note: Keep your front torso long and your left heel grounded.*

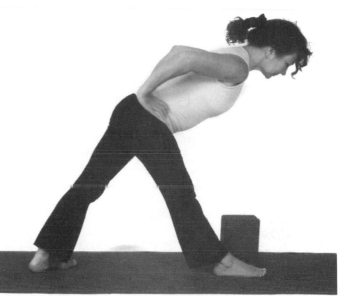

4 Exhale and turn to the right. Reach down with your left hand and press on the end of the block. Inhale and stretch your right arm toward the ceiling. Hold for 30 seconds to 1 minute. *Note: Be sure, as you turn, not to shorten your front torso. Hold the right-leg hip in (to the pelvis) and back (toward the wall behind you), and lean back against your scapulas.*

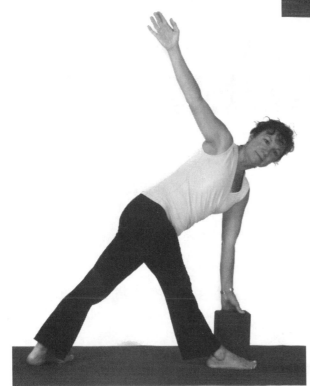

To Come Up: Exhale, release the twist, and inhale your torso back to upright.

Extended Side Angle Pose

Perform to the right then repeat to the left

Utthita parshvakonasana (oo-TEE-tah parsh-vah-cone-AHS-anna)
utthita = extended; parshva = side, flank; kona = angle

When performing this pose, the tendency is to focus the "extension" or stretch on the topside of the torso (the side between the back leg and the top arm). It might be more appropriate to name this pose Extended *Sides* Angle; that's because you want to try to extend the underside of the torso as much as the topside.

1 Spread your feet 3 to 4 feet apart. Turn your right foot out 90 degrees, your left foot in 30 degrees. Set your block on one side outside your right foot. Rest your hands on your hips.
Note: Make sure your heels are aligned and your left heel is actively pressed to the floor (or against the corner of the room) to anchor the pose.

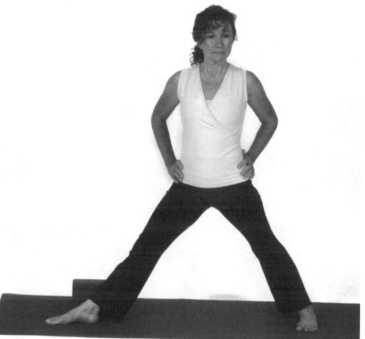

2 With your pelvis turned slightly to the right, turn your upper torso (rib cage) to the left. Exhale and quickly bend your right knee over your right ankle.
Note: If your thigh doesn't drop quite parallel to the floor, try widening your stance by a few inches.

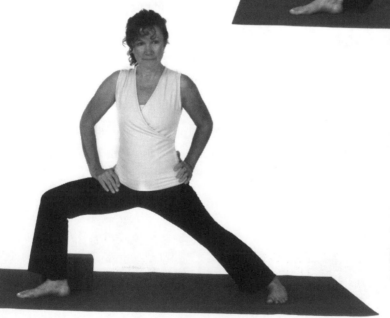

BENEFITS

Strengthens and stretches the legs, knees, and ankles; stretches the groins, spine, waist, chest and lungs, and shoulders.

TIP

You can also perform this pose with the bottom arm and hand in front of, and pushing back against, the bent-knee thigh.

CHALLENGE YOURSELF

When you bend down, lay the underside of your torso flat on the front-leg thigh.

3 Exhale and bend over so the right side of your torso nears your right thigh. Turn your upper torso slightly to the right, reach your right hand down onto the block. *Note: Actively press your right knee out against your right arm.*

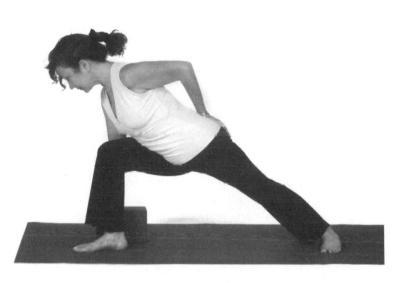

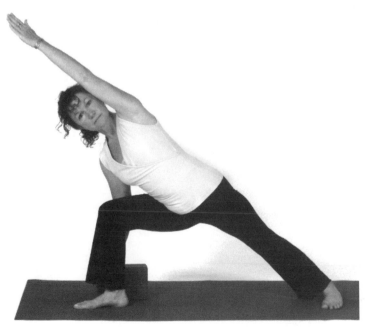

4 Turn your upper torso back to the left; inhale and extend your left arm over your head just behind your left ear so that it is parallel to your spine. Stay for 30 seconds to 1 minute.

To Come Up: Inhale and lift your torso back to upright by pressing down through your back heel and reaching up through your top arm.

Virabhadra's Pose I

Commonly called Warrior Pose, variation 1

Virabhadrasana I (veer-ah-bah-DRAHS-anna)
Virabhadra = a fierce warrior, an emanation and emissary of Shiva, fondly nicknamed the "Monster of Destruction." He (it?) had a thousand heads and eyes, a thousand feet, countless weapons, and enormous tusks protruding from his mouth. He wore snakes and lion and tiger skins, and dripped with blood. In short, not someone you want to meet in a dark alley.

1 Spread your feet 3 to 4 feet apart. Turn your right foot out 90 degrees, place your left heel on a sandbag and turn it in about 45 to 60 degrees. Rest your hands on your hips. *Note: Make sure your heels are aligned and your left heel is pressed firmly to the bag to anchor the pose.*

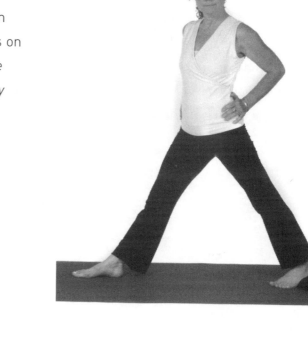

2 With an exhale, turn your torso to the right as close to 90 degrees as is comfortable while keeping your left leg straight. *Note: Lengthen your tail toward the floor and lift your pubis toward your navel.*

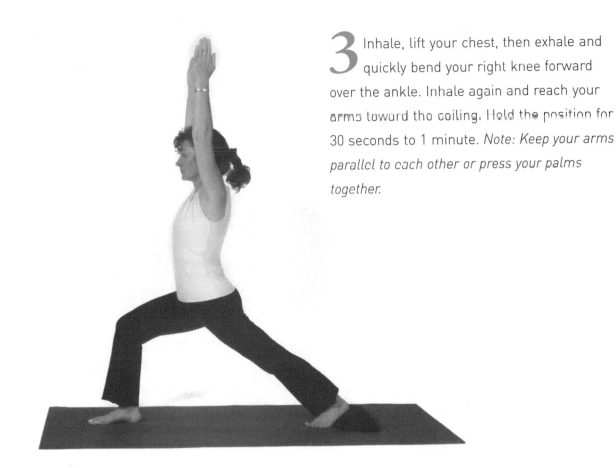

3 Inhale, lift your chest, then exhale and quickly bend your right knee forward over the ankle. Inhale again and reach your arms toward the ceiling. Hold the position for 30 seconds to 1 minute. *Note: Keep your arms parallel to each other or press your palms together.*

To Come Up: On the inhale, press your back heel firmly and lift through your arms, straightening your front knee.

Virabhadra's Pose II

Commonly called Warrior Pose, variation 2

Virabhadrasana II (veer-ah-bah-DRAHS-anna)

Although he had a demonic appearance, Virabhadra's true nature was "full of wisdom, detachment, sovereignty, asceticism, truth, patience, fortitude, lordship, and self-knowledge" (from Stella Kramrisch, Speaking of Shiva, 323).

1 Spread your feet 3 to 4 feet apart. Turn your right foot out 90 degrees, your left foot in about 30 degrees. Rest your hands here on your hips.

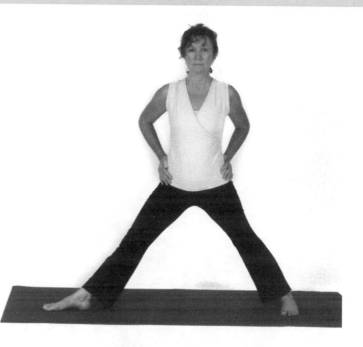

2 Exhale and bend your right knee over your right ankle until your shin is perpendicular to the floor. Inhale and raise your arms parallel to the floor. *Note: Your torso will tend to lean over the right thigh. Try to keep your shoulders aligned over your pelvis so that your spine stays perpendicular to the floor.*

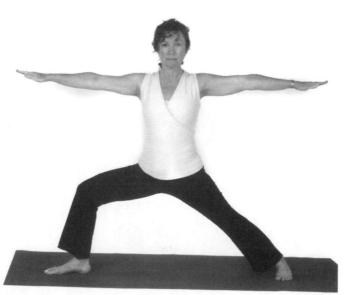

46

BENEFITS

Strengthens and stretches the legs and ankles; stretches the groins, chest and lungs, and shoulders; and increases endurance.

CAUTION

If you have a neck injury, don't turn your head to look at the front hand—simply look straight ahead.

TIP

To increase the stretch of your arms, turn your palms toward the ceiling. Reach actively through your fingers. Without losing the rotation of your upper arms, turn your palms from the wrists to face the floor.

CHALLENGE YOURSELF

For most beginners, the bent-knee thigh is slightly above parallel to the floor. See if you can gradually lower the thigh to a parallel position.

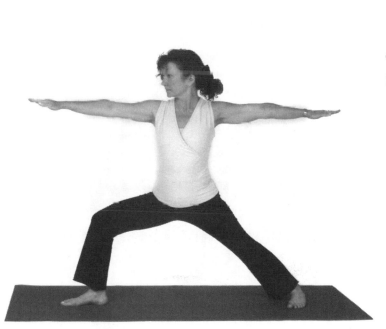

3 Turn your head to the right and gaze at your fingertips. Stay for 30 seconds to 1 minute.

To Come Up: Inhale and straighten your front knee, pulling yourself up by reaching out through your back arm.

Half Moon Pose

Ardha chandrasana (ar-dah chan-DRAHS-anna)
ardha = half; chandra = glittering, shining (like the gods), but usually rendered as "moon"

Where's the half moon? Look at the model in the final picture: in your imagination, draw a half circle from the standing foot to the raised foot to the raised arm, then a straight line down from the raised arm through to the standing foot. See it now?

Perform to the right then repeat to the left

1 Stand with your back to a wall, one leg's length away. Place a yoga block about a foot in front of your left foot. Exhale and bend forward.

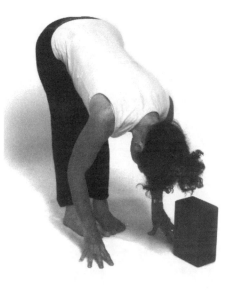

2 Place your left hand on the block, right hand on the floor. Inhale, swing your right leg up parallel to the floor, and press your foot against the wall. *Note: Point your toes to the floor and keep your standing leg perpendicular to the floor.*

47

BENEFITS

Strengthens the ankles, thighs, buttocks, and spine; stretches the groins, hamstrings, calves, shoulders, chest, and spine; and improves your sense of balance.

CAUTION

The standing knee in Half Moon tends to roll in, a possible cause of strain. Be sure to keep the "eye" of the kneecap looking straight ahead.

CHALLENGE YOURSELF

Half Moon Pose is normally a free-standing pose. To increase the challenge, take the raised foot slightly away from the wall. Balance mostly on the standing leg and press the bottom hand lightly against the yoga block.

3 On your next inhale, raise your right hand up to your right hip. Then as you exhale, turn your upper torso to the right and pivot your right foot outward on its heel until the inner foot is parallel to the floor. *Note: Press your right heel actively against the wall. Look straight out.*

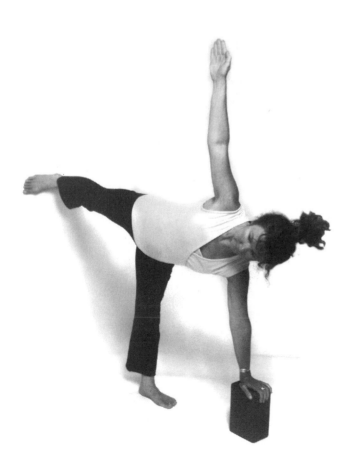

4 Move the block in your left hand forward up to about a foot. Inhale and extend your right arm toward the ceiling. Stay for 30 seconds to 1 minute.

To Come Up: Turn your torso back to face the floor, and exhale back to the standing forward bend.

Intense Wide-Leg Forward Bend

Prasarita padottanasana (pra-sa-REE-tah pah-doh-tahn-AHS-anna)
prasarita = stretched out, expanded, spread, with outstretched limbs
pada = foot; ud = intense; tan = to stretch or extend

This pose is in what I call the "ut family" of poses along with Intense Stretch Pose, Intense Side Stretch Pose and Intense-Stretch-of-the-West Pose. While still powerful stretches, my variation here makes them a little less "ut" (intense).

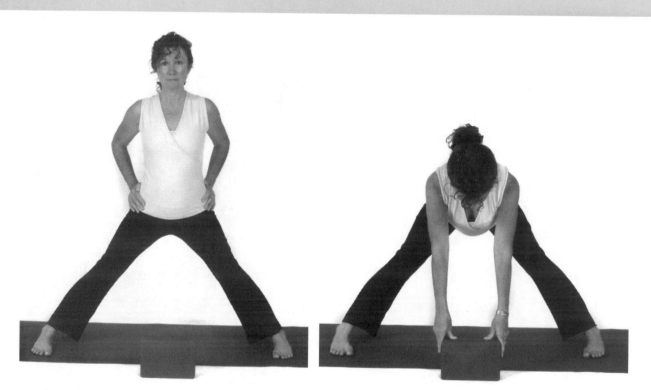

1 Place your yoga block on its side directly in front of you. Spread your feet 3 to 4 feet apart. Rest your hands on your hips, inhale, and lift your chest. *Note: Make sure your feet are parallel, the outer edges pressing firmly into the floor.*

2 Exhale and tip your torso forward from the hip joints until it is parallel to the floor. Press your fingertips on the block directly below your shoulders.

BENEFITS

Strengthens and stretches the inner and back legs and spine; tones the abdominal organs; and calms the brain.

CAUTION

Avoid the full forward bend (as described in step 4) if you have any serious lower back problems.

TIP

If your inner arches sag, lift your toes away from the floor and purposely shift some of your weight to the outside edges of your feet. Then, without losing the lift of your arches, soften your toes back to the floor.

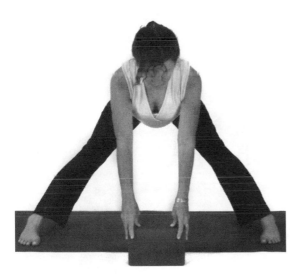

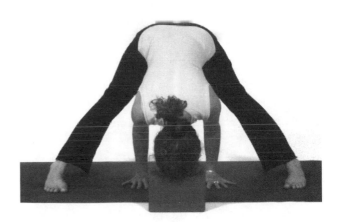

3 Slightly arch your back by lifting your sitting bones and stretching your manubrium forward. Gaze straight ahead or down at the floor. Take a few breaths in this position.

4 Then with an exhale, lower your torso into a full forward bend, placing your forehead on the block. Stay for 30 seconds to 2 minutes. *Note: Keeping your arms parallel, elbows bent, walk your hands back between your feet.*

To Come Up: Place your hands on your hips, lengthen your front torso, and lift your torso with an inhale back to upright. Walk your feet together.

Intense Stretch Pose

Commonly called Standing Forward Bend

Uttanasana (oot-tan-AHS-ahna)

ut = intense; tan = to stretch or extend. The Sanskrit verb tan *is related to the Latin*
tendere, *"to stretch, extend." This word is the root of many familiar English words, such*
as tend, tent, and tense; many "-tend" words, like attend, contend, and pretend; and many
"-tain" words, like contain, maintain, obtain, retain, and sustain.

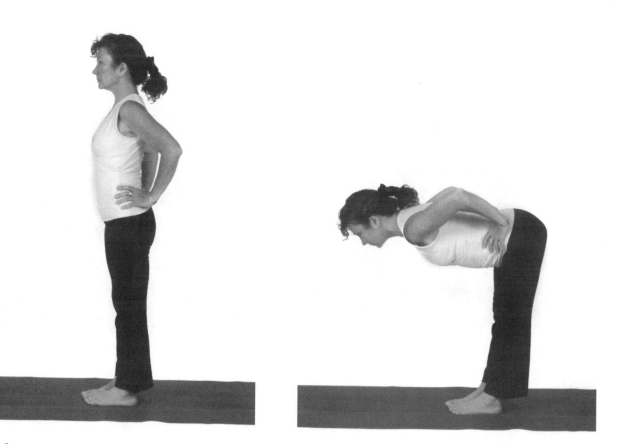

1 Stand in Mountain, with your feet parallel to each other and a few inches apart. Rest your hands on your hips.

2 Inhale, lift your chest, then exhale and tip your torso forward. *Note: As always in a forward bend, move from your hip joints, not your belly.*

BENEFITS

Stretches the hamstrings, calves, and hips; strengthens the thighs; and calms the brain.

CAUTION

Avoid this pose if you have a serious back injury, or perform it only with bent knees.

CHALLENGE YOURSELF

To increase the stretch on the backs of your legs, stand with the balls of your feet lifted on a sand bag or thick book.

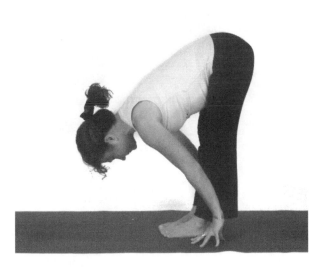

3 On an inhale, slightly lift and lengthen your front torso. Then on the following exhale, dive deeper into the forward bend. Stay for 30 seconds to 2 minutes. *Note: Let your head hang heavily, imagining that it's rooted deep in your upper back. This pose is often used as a resting pose between the other standing poses.*

To Come Up: Bring your hands back to your hips, lengthen your front torso, and lift up with an inhale.

Intense Side Stretch Pose

Parshvottanasana (parsh-voh-tahn-AHS-anna)
parshva = side, flank; ud = intense; tan = to stretch or extend

Perform to the right then repeat to the left

Intense Side Stretch Pose is typically performed with the palms pressed together behind the back torso. Here, though, we'll have you rest them on yoga blocks to help maintain your balance during the stretch.

1 Spread your feet 3 to 4 feet apart. Turn your right foot out 90 degrees, your left foot in about 45 to 60 degrees. Set two blocks on either side of your right foot. Rest your hands on your hips. *Note: Make sure your heels are aligned and your left heel is actively pressed to the floor (or against the corner of the room) to anchor the pose.*

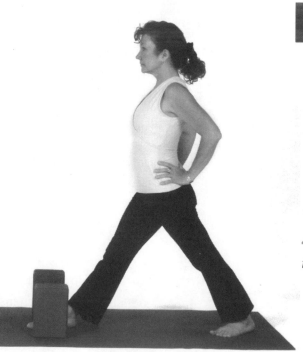

2 With an exhale, twist your torso to the right. *Note: Lengthen your tail toward the floor and lift your pubis toward your navel.*

BENEFITS

Stretches the spine, shoulders, wrists, hips, and hamstrings; strengthens the legs; and improves posture and your sense of balance.

CAUTION

In this pose, the forward-leg hip tends to ride up, unbalancing the pelvis and compressing the forward-leg side of the spine. If this happens, bend the forward knee slightly, align the back of the pelvis parallel to the floor, then slowly re-straighten the knee.

CHALLENGE YOURSELF

To increase the challenge in this pose, lower your torso past the parallel position. Bring your chest close to the front of the forward leg. Be careful, though: if you do this, to keep the front torso long, don't round forward from your belly.

3 Exhale and tip your torso forward until it's approximately parallel to the floor. Reach down and press your hands onto the yoga blocks. Stay for 30 seconds to 1 minute. *Note: Press your right-leg hip firmly into the torso and draw it back toward the wall behind you. Adjust the front of your pelvis so it's parallel to the floor.*

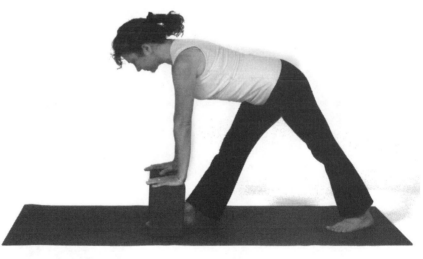

To Come Up: Inhale and lift up with a long front torso.

55

Powerful Pose

Sometimes called Chair Pose

Utkatasana (oot-kah-TAHS-anna)

utkata = powerful, fierce

While this pose does indeed look like the practitioner is sitting on a chair (and thus is often called Chair Pose), remember that *utkata* has nothing to do with a chair. The little particle *ud* in this word (which becomes *ut* when combined with *kata*) means "up, over, above," and implies superiority in place, rank, or power.

1 Stand in Mountain. With an inhale, sweep your arms out to your sides and up, perpendicular to the floor. *Note: Keep your arms parallel and move them as close together as is comfortable, even pressing your palms together if you can do so without tensing the neck and shoulders.*

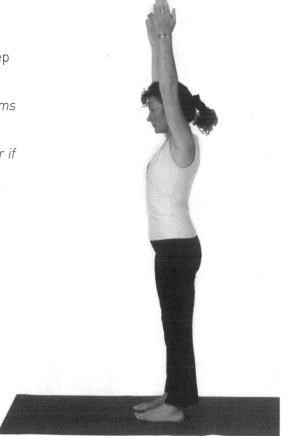

BENEFITS

Strengthens the ankles, thighs, and spine; and stretches shoulders and chest.

CAUTION

The tail bone in this pose tends to Donald-Duck-tail out, compressing the lower spine. Be sure to keep your tail pressing slightly down and forward to lengthen the lower back.

TIP

The thighs tend to splay in this pose. To keep your thighs parallel and at the same time strengthen them, squeeze a block placed between your thighs slightly above your knees.

2 Inhale, lift your chest, then exhale and bend your knees until your thighs are nearly parallel to the floor. Stay for 30 seconds to 1 minute. *Note: Your knees should push out over your feet and your torso will lean slightly forward. Lengthen your tail bone toward the floor. Be sure not to overly arch your lower back. Hold your inner thighs parallel to each other.*

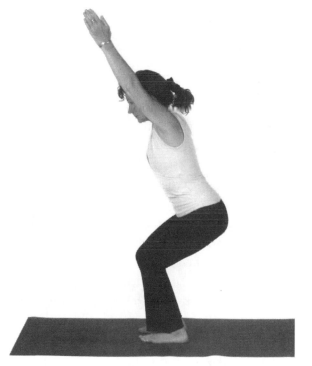

To Come Up: Inhale, reach through your arms, and straighten your knees. Then exhale your hands to your sides and return to Mountain.

belly poses

In this section, you'll strengthen and stretch the belly. If someone asked you to point to your belly, you would probably point to the general vicinity of your belly button; but this area is better thought of as the front belly. The belly actually includes the entire cylindrical area between the bell-shaped rib case and the bowl-shaped pelvis.

Three different belly muscles are of interest here. The first is the rectus abdominis (RA), the long muscle that runs vertically downward from the middle ribs and lower sternum to the pubis. You can easily run your fingers along the RA. When standing upright, contraction of this muscle helps to bend your torso forward (flexion); in a back bend, the RA relaxes and stretches.

The second belly muscle is the psoas (PS), and it is actually a pair of muscles. You might not think of the PS pair as belly muscles, but they are, located (for the most part) at the back belly. If you could remove the front of your belly, scoop out the organs, and look into the belly cavity (and at the front of the spine),

you'd see that your PS pair forms a long inverted V. The apex of this inverted V is at the lower (lumbar) spine; the tips of its two legs (after they sweep through the back pelvis and forward over the pubis) attach to the tops of the inner femurs. When you contract one of your PS muscles in the upright position, and hold your torso steady, the same-side thigh will lift (or flex); every time you take a step forward when walking, you contract your PS. If you fix your feet to the floor and contract both PS muscles together, your torso will bend forward (flex). In a back bend, these muscles relax and stretch.

The third belly muscle (actually, another muscle pair) is the abdominal obliques (OB) (to be accurate, there is an oblique exterior oblique muscle and an interior oblique muscle). They're located on the sides of the belly, between the rib case and the pelvis. When standing upright, contraction of either one of this muscle pair bends your torso to the side (lateral flexion) or twists your torso right or left.

PROP: *You'll need a block for the poses in this section.*

CHALLENGE YOURSELF

To increase the challenge in this pose,
perform it without the block support.

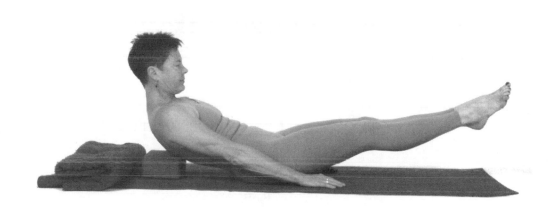

3 With another exhale, lift your right leg away from the floor until the tip of the big toe is level with your right eye. Hold for 10 to 15 seconds, then release. Repeat with your left leg for the same length of time. Finally lift both legs for 10 to 15 seconds, breathing smoothly.

To Come Up: Release your leg(s) to the floor with an exhale. Then roll off the block to one side with another exhale.

Twist-around-the-belly Pose

Perform to the left then repeat to the right

Also called Reclining Twist

Jathara Parivartanasana (jah-TAR-ah par-ee-var-tan-AHS-anna)
jathara = belly or womb; parivartana = turning round, revolving

In the full pose, the legs are extended toward the outstretched hands and the feet lifted a few inches off the floor. Here we'll perform the pose with the knees bent and the legs resting on the floor.

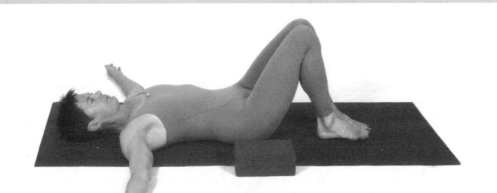

1 Lie on your back with your knees bent, feet on the floor, and arms stretched out to your sides, parallel to the line of your shoulders. Place a yoga block 1 foot outside your right thigh.

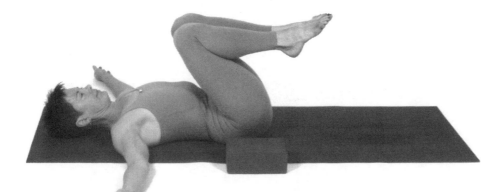

2 Exhale and draw your thighs to your torso. *Note: Maintain this sharp angle between the thighs and torso for the entire exercise.*

BENEFITS

Reclining Twist tones the abdominal obliques (OB), stretches the chest and shoulders, relaxes the lower back, and improves digestion.

CAUTIONS

If your shoulder lifts off the floor (on the side you're twisting away from), be sure not to force it back to the floor. Turning your head away from the twist is acceptable, but be sure not to strain your neck; if you feel strain, look straight up at the ceiling.

CHALLENGE YOURSELF

Once you're comfortably in the pose, you can increase the stretch by removing the block and swinging your legs till they rest on the ground. Try lifting your feet a few inches ways off the floor and hold them there for 5 to 10 seconds.

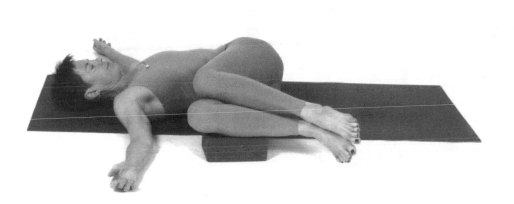

3 As you twist, continue to look up at the ceiling. Exhale and swing your bent legs to the right and down onto the yoga block. Hold for 1 to 2 minutes. *Note: As your pelvis turns right, turn your rib case back to the left and reach actively through your left arm.*

To Come Up: Inhale to return to neutral.

Upward Extended Legs Pose

Repeat 5 to 15 times as you get stronger

Also called Leg Swings

Urdhva Prasarita Padasana (erd-vah pra-sa-REE-tah pod-AHS-anna)
urdhva = upward; prasarita = stretched out, expanded, spread, with outstretched limbs; pada = foot. The Sanksrit pada is distantly related to the Latin ped, "foot," the root of many English words such as pedestrian, pedal, podium, and—yes—octopus. You'll also find this word in Prasarita Padottanasana (page 50) and Supta Padangushtasana (page 82).

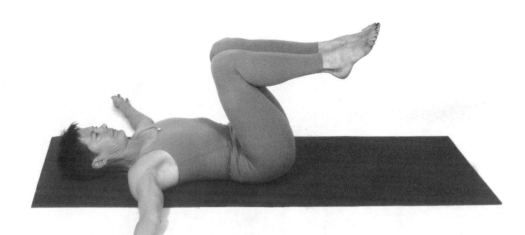

1 Lie on your back with your knees bent, feet on the floor, and arms stretched alongside your torso, palms pressing into the floor. Exhale, keeping your knees bent, and lift your feet off the floor until your thighs are perpendicular to the floor. *Note: Your knees should be directly over your hips.*

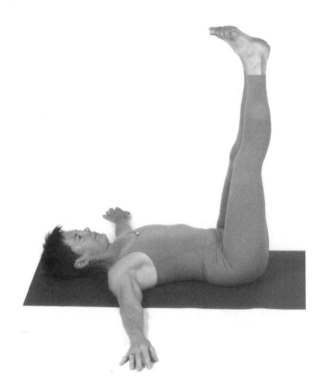

2 Inhale and extend your feet upward so that your legs are perpendicular to the floor. *Note: Don't point your toes; press your heels actively toward the ceiling.*

BENEFIT

Strengthening the psoas (PS) pair.

CAUTIONS

Avoid this pose if you have a lower back injury or herniated disk.

TIPS

Keep your throat, jaw, and eyes soft. Since this is a PS exercise, your rectus abdominis (RA) should be firm and relatively flat, not hard and rounded.

CHALLENGE YOURSELF

To increase the challenge in this pose, reach your arms overhead and lay them on the floor, palms up.

3 Exhale and swing your legs down until you feel your lower back begin to lift away from the floor and your belly harden. Hold. Inhale. *Note: How far your legs move will depend on the strength of your psoas pair. Eventually you'll be able to lower your heels to within an inch or so of the floor.*

4 Exhale and swing your legs back to vertical. *Note: Be sure to move your legs down and up only on an exhale; hold them steady during the inhale.*

To Come Up: After completing your rounds, with your legs vertical, bend your knees and, with an exhale, float your feet softly to the floor.

arm-strength poses

In this section, you will strengthen the wrists and arms. Strength poses are frequently the bugaboo of beginners. Don't despair! Practice regularly and remember what Krishna tells Arjuna in the Bhagavad-Gita: No effort is ever wasted.

The two poses in this section both begin in Downward Facing Dog Pose (page 24).

PROPS: *You'll need a blanket or two for the first pose, and, optionally, a wall for the second.*

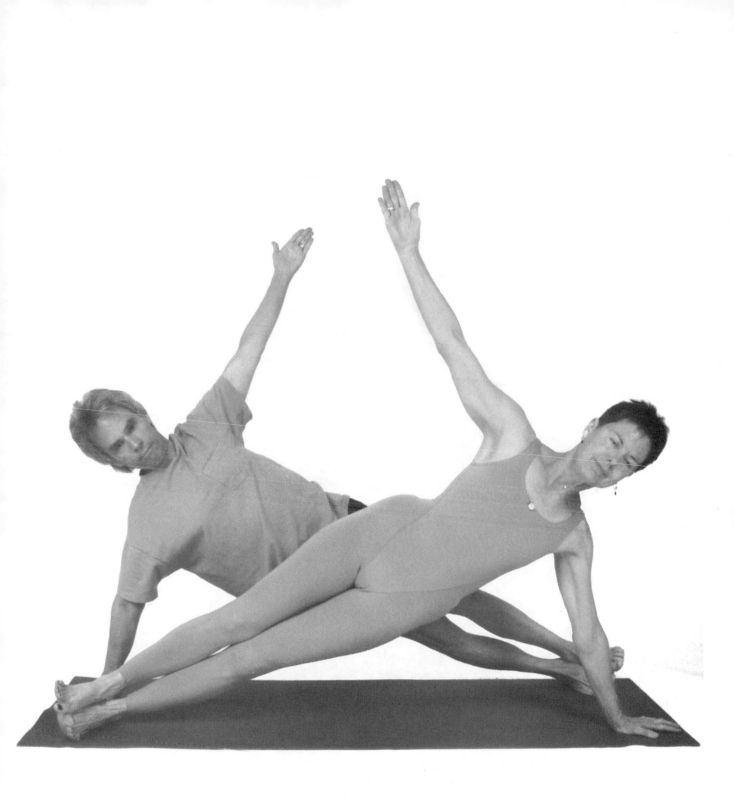

Four-Limb Staff Pose

Chaturanga Dandasana (chaht-tour-ANG-ah don-DAHS-anna)
chaturanga = four limbs (chatur = four; anga = limb); danda = staff

The "four limbs" here refers to this pose's four supports: the two hands and (the balls of the) two feet. The "staff" refers to the spine, the central support of the body (for more on the spine, see Staff Pose, page 74).

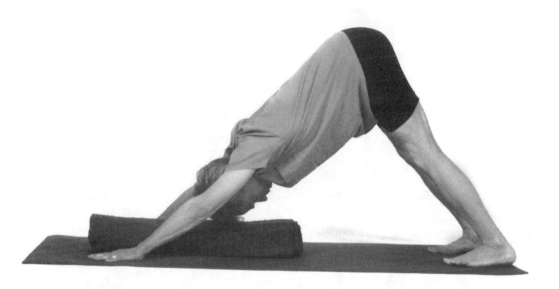

1 Begin in Downward Facing Dog. Position a rolled-up blanket measuring 6 inches thick and 2 feet long below your torso.

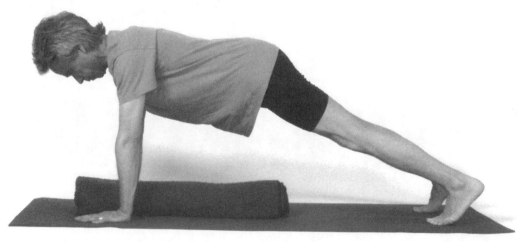

2 Inhale and swing your torso forward, aligning your shoulders over your hands. *Note: Your arms should be perpendicular to the floor and your torso parallel to the floor. This is called Plank.*

BENEFITS

Strengthens the arms, wrists, and front belly.

CAUTIONS

Avoid this pose if you have any serious shoulder or wrist injury.

CHALLENGE YOURSELF

Remove the blanket and perform the pose with your hands and knees serving as supports. Or try the full pose with your hands and the balls of your feet serving as supports. In these, lower your torso and legs to within a few inches of the floor. Be sure not to let the pelvis sag as you did on the blanket support; press your tail toward your pubis and firm your thighs, lifting them toward the ceiling.

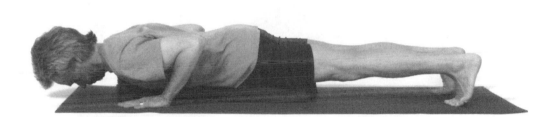

3 Exhale and slowly, bending your elbows, lower your torso and legs onto the support. *Note: Try not to simply collapse downward—lower yourself with a modicum of control.*

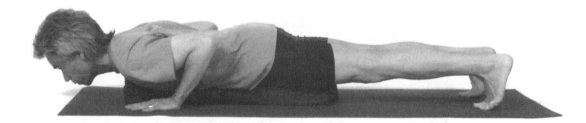

4 Rest your torso and thighs as lightly as possible on the support. Look forward. Hold for 15 to 30 seconds. *Note: Press your tail toward your pubis and imagine your thighs lifting away from the support. Keep your upper arms in, parallel to the sides of your torso.*

To Come Up: With an exhale, push back to Downward Facing Dog.

Vashishtha's Pose

Vashishthasana (vah-shish-TAHS-anna)
Vashishtha = literally means "most excellent, best, richest." This is the name of several well-known ancient sages. Maybe the most famous is said to be the owner of Nandini ("delight"), the so-called "cow of plenty," which grants his every wish (thus he's the "richest").

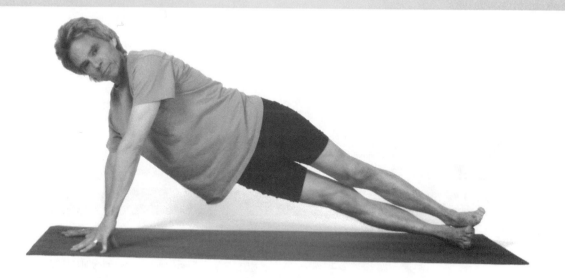

1 Begin in Plank. Shift to the outside edge of your right foot, then stack your left foot on top of the right.

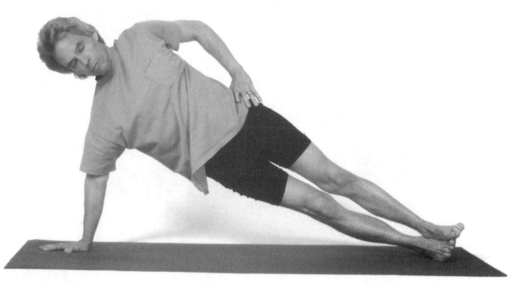

2 Swing your left hand onto your left hip and turn your torso to the left. *Note: Make sure that your supporting hand is a few inches forward of its shoulder so that your arm is slightly angled (and not perpendicular) relative to the floor.*

BENEFITS

Strengthens the arms and wrists, belly, and legs; and improves your sense of balance.

CAUTIONS

Avoid this pose if you have serious wrist, elbow, or shoulder injuries.

TIP

If you find it difficult to balance in this pose, perform Downward Facing Dog with your heels lifted against a wall. Then when you turn into Vashishtha's Pose, press your soles against the wall.

CHALLENGE YOURSELF

Try the full version of this pose by raising the top leg perpendicular to the supporting leg and holding its big toe between the index and middle finger of the top-side hand.

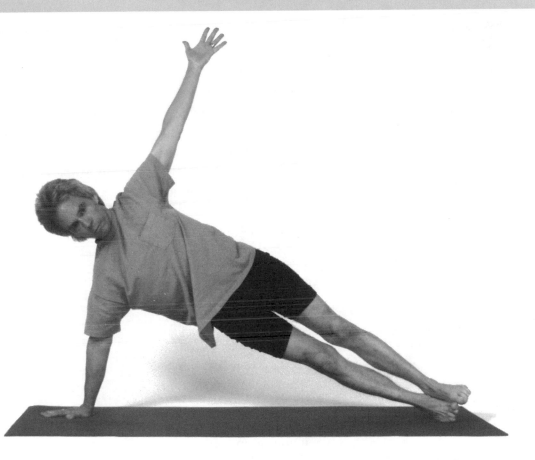

3 Raise your left hand off your hip and aim it up in a line parallel to the line of your shoulders (and not perpendicular to the floor). Stay for 20 seconds to 1 minute. *Note: Your body (except your arms) should form one long diagonal line from your crown to your heels. Don't sag your pelvis toward the floor or lift it out of the diagonal toward the ceiling. Also keep your tail pressed slightly forward toward your pubis so that your buttocks don't stick out.*

To Come Up: Return with an exhale to Downward Facing Dog.

sitting poses and forward bends

In this section, you'll do sitting poses and forward bends. Like their standing counterparts (for example, Intense Stretch Pose; see page 52), these poses provide an enormous stretch for the muscles at the backs of the legs, especially the hamstrings on the back thighs. And therein lies the rub.

These three muscles (three on each leg) run between the sitting bones and the two lower leg bones (tibia and fibula). Whenever you want to tip the pelvis into a forward bend, the hamstrings must release and lengthen; if they don't, you won't get very far forward—unless you bend your knees. But bending the knees, to a certain extent, defeats the purpose of the pose, which is to stretch the back legs.

Most beginners have tight hamstrings, and consequently their forward bends are restricted. And when hamstrings reach their limit in a forward bend, beginners tend to cheat: they continue the movement by rounding farther forward from the belly.

This shortens the front of the torso and humps the back torso, risking lumbar strain. Always remember to move into a forward bend from the hip joints, never the belly. Keep the front of your torso—between the pubis and navel, and navel and sternum—as long as possible.

Sit in Staff (see page 74) as the starting and ending point of all the sitting forward bends (that is, Head-to-Knee, Seated Wide-Leg, and Intense Stretch-of-the-West poses), as well as Cow Face and Bound Angle poses.

TIP

When you sit on the floor for Staff and ready yourself to either sit upright or bend forward (in Easy, Cow Face, Bound Angle, Head-to-Knee, Seated Wide-Leg, and Intense Stretch-of-the-West poses), your pelvis should be in a neutral position. That means that the line of your waist is parallel, and your torso is relatively perpendicular to the floor. Most beginners need to sit up on a thickly folded blanket to achieve this alignment. Be careful: If you move into a forward bend with your pelvis in a backward-tilting position (with your tail closer to the floor than your pubis is), you risk straining your lower back.

PROPS: For the forward bends, you'll need a blanket, a block, and a strap.

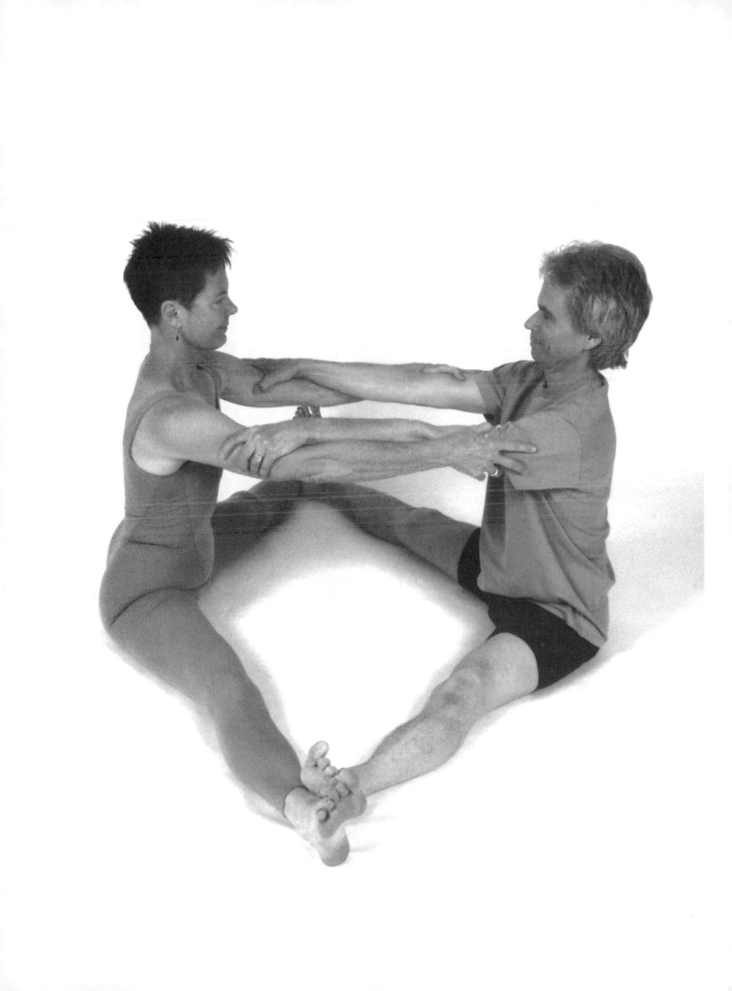

Staff Pose

Dandasana (dahn-DAHS-anna)
danda = staff (as a symbol of power and sovereignty), stick, rod

The staff refers to the spine, the central support of the body. Our spine is also called the Meru-danda, the "staff of Meru," an allusion to the mythical Mount Meru that serves as the "hub" of the Hindu universe.

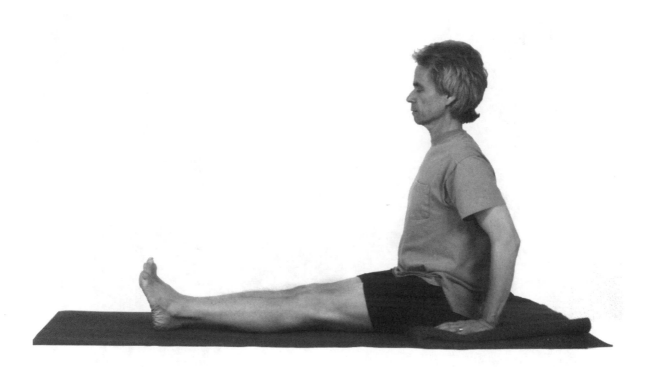

1 Sit on a thickly folded blanket with your legs straight out in front of your torso. Push actively through your heels and the bases of your big toes, but don't lift your heels off the floor. Turn your upper thighs slightly inward, and lengthen your tail toward the floor. Press your palms (fingers pointing forward) on the floor beside your hips.

BENEFITS

Staff strengthens the back muscles and thighs; stretches the chest; and improves posture.

CHALLENGE YOURSELF

To increase the challenge In this pose, inhale and raise your arms perpendicular to the floor. You can keep your arms parallel to each other, or join the palms. Hold for a few seconds, then release your arms with an exhale.

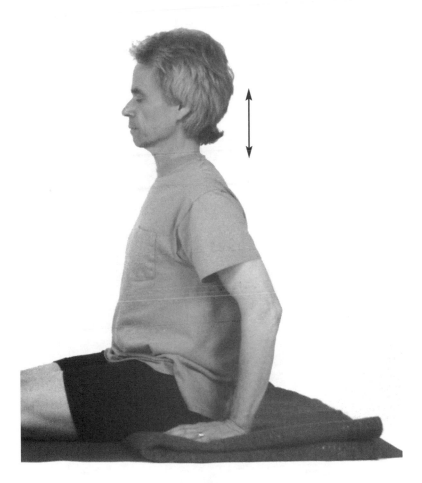

2 Lift the base of your skull away from the back of your neck to balance your head on top of your spine. At the same time, draw the crook of your throat diagonally toward the top of your spine to bring the whole head in line with the spine. Press your scapulae and your sacrum firmly against your back torso, and lift the top of your sternum toward the ceiling. Hold for 1 to 3 minutes.

To Come Up: Release with an exhale.

Hero Pose

Virasana (veer-AHS-anna)

vira = man, hero, chief (compare Latin vir, *"man," the root of English words virile and virtue)*

In the full version of this pose, the buttocks rest on the floor between the feet. Here your buttocks will rest on a block placed between your feet.

1 Kneel with your thighs perpendicular to the floor, inner knees touching. Your feet are slightly wider than your hips. Set your yoga block between your feet.
Note: See that your toes point straight back, not out to the sides.

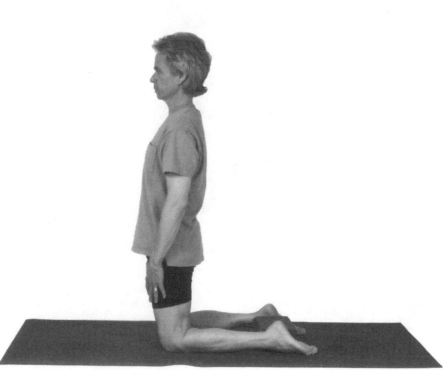

BENEFITS

Hero stretches the thighs, knees, and ankles.

CAUTIONS

Avoid this pose if you have any serious knee or ankle injuries.

TIP

Some beginners find this pose very painful on their ankles. If you find this to be a problem, sit in the pose with a rolled-up towel under your ankles.

2 Sit back slowly onto the block. Turn your thighs inward with your hands. Lift your chest as your lengthen your tail down toward the floor. Then lay your hands on your thighs, palms down. Hold for 30 seconds. *Note: Keep your thighs parallel to each other; don't allow your knees to splay out to the sides. If you prefer, you can stack your hands on your lap, palms up. Gradually over several weeks, increase the time you spend in Hero until you can comfortably sit for 5 minutes.*

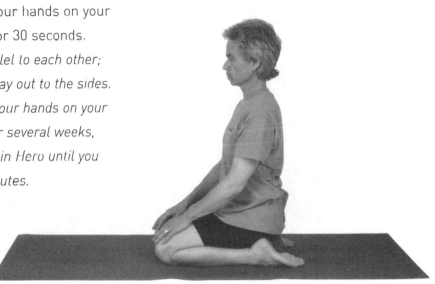

To Come Up: Lift up and move the block off to one side. Press your hands against the floor, cross your ankles below your buttocks, then sit back on the floor so that your crossed ankles are now in front of your pelvis. Stretch one leg at a time out to your side so that you end up in a wide-leg sitting position, then slide the legs together back to Staff.

Cow Face Pose

Gomukhasana (go-moo-KAHS-anna)

go = cow (Sanskrit go *is a distant relative of the English word "cow"); mukha = face*

Why is this pose named Cow Face? If you can do this pose in front of a mirror, look at your crossed legs. See the cow's lips? Then look at your arms. See the ears, one up, one down? Moo.

In the full version of this pose, the hands are hooked behind the back. Here we'll use a strap to secure the hands in place.

Repeat with legs and arms reversed for the same length of time

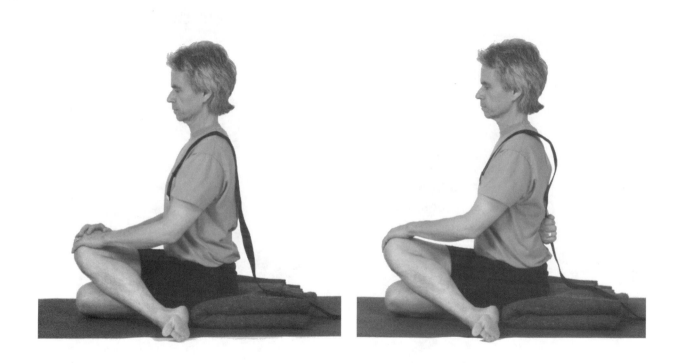

1 Sit on a blanket with your legs crossed, right leg on top. *Note: To safely cross your legs, bend your knees and set your feet on the floor. Slide your left foot under your right leg and position your heel outside your right hip. Then stack your right knee on top of the left, with your right heel on the floor outside your left hip.*

2 Drape your yoga strap over your left shoulder. Exhale your right arm around behind your back, and grasp the yoga strap in your right hand. *Note: Make sure to draw your right arm into the hollow of your lower back, parallel to your waist.*

BENEFITS

Cow Face stretches the ankles, hips, thighs, shoulders, the backs of the upper arms, and chest.

CAUTIONS

Avoid the leg position in this pose if you have any serious knee or ankle problems; avoid the arm position if you have any serious shoulder problems.

CHALLENGE YOURSELF

If you have the flexibility in your shoulders and armpits, you can try to hook your fingers behind your back. Actively pull the hands apart (but don't actually release the grip), and lift your chest.

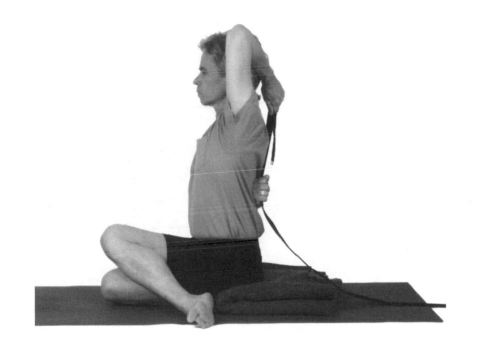

3 Holding the front end of the strap in your left hand, inhale your left arm straight up. Exhale and bend your elbow. Walk your hands along the strap toward each other as close as you comfortably can. Hold for 1 to 2 minutes. *Note. Keep your right elbow close to your side and your left arm close to your ear.*

To Come Up: Release your arms with an exhale and uncross your legs back to Staff.

Bound Angle Pose

Also called the Cobbler's Pose

Baddha Konasana (bah-dah cone-AHS-anna)

baddha = bound; kona = angle

In India, cobblers sit in this position for hours, repairing shoes with their tools held between their feet.

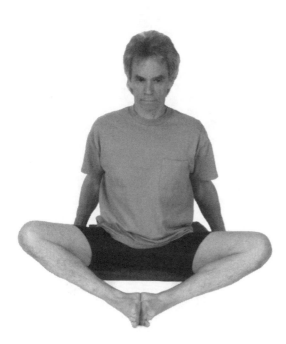

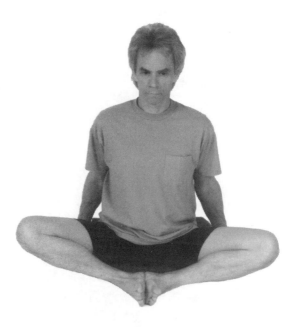

1 From Staff Pose, exhale, bend your knees, and touch your soles together.

2 Draw your heels toward your perineum as close as you comfortably can. Soften your inner groins and release your knees toward the floor. *Note: Let your knees drop down—do not forcefully press them down.*

BENEFITS

Bound Angle stretches the inner thighs, groins, and knees. Traditional texts say that this pose destroys disease and gets rid of fatigue.

CAUTIONS

If you have a groin or knee injury, only practice this pose with your outer thighs supported on thickly folded blankets.

CHALLENGE YOURSELF

To increase the stretch on your inner thighs, lean your torso slightly forward. Be sure to keep the front of your torso long. Bend from your hips, not your belly.

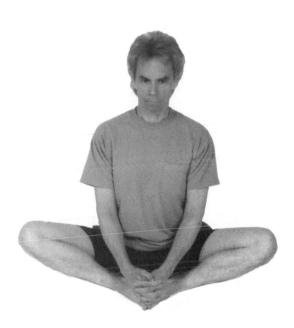

3 Clasp your hands around your toes, but press the little toes against the floor. Hold for 1 to 5 minutes. *Note: If you can't easily reach your feet, grip your ankles or even your shins.*

To Come Up: Inhale, draw your thighs together, and stretch your legs back out to Staff.

Reclining Big Toe Pose

Supta Padangushtasana (soup-tah pod-ang-goosh-TAHS-anna)
supta = lying down, reclining; pada = foot; angushta = big toe

In the full version of this pose, the big toe of the raised foot is gripped by the same-side hand (and so the name). Here we'll use a strap to hold the raised foot.

Perform with the right leg then repeat with the left

1 Lie on your back, both legs extended along the floor. Exhale, bend your right knee, and draw your thigh into your belly. Wrap the strap around your sole.

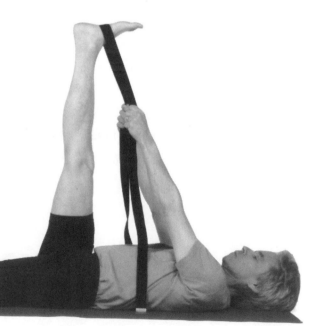

2 With an inhale, push through your right heel and straighten your leg perpendicular to the floor. *Note: Press your shoulder blades evenly against the floor. Spread your clavicles. Press your left thigh heavily against the floor and push actively through your left heel.*

BENEFITS

Reclining Big Toe stretches the hips, thighs, hamstrings, and calves; and strengthens the thighs.

CAUTIONS

Be sure that your head rests comfortably on the floor. If the back of your head is pulled down and your chin juts up toward the ceiling, rest your head on a thickly folded blanket.

TIP

If you have difficulty keeping your floor leg active, lie so that you can press the floor-leg heel against a wall.

CHALLENGE YOURSELF

Position a block on one face just outside your right hip. Exhale, gently pull your right leg out to the side, and lower it onto the block. Hold for a few seconds, then inhale and draw your leg back to vertical. Repeat with the left leg.

3 Holding the strap lightly, walk your hands up the strap until your arms are fully extended. Hold for 1 to 3 minutes. *Note: If the back of your neck shortens when you raise your leg, support your head on a thickly folded blanket. Be sure not to use the strap to PULL your leg into a deeper stretch.*

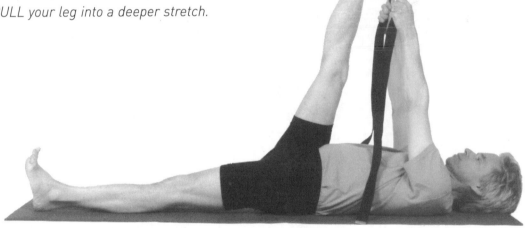

To Come Up: Release the raised leg with an exhale back to the floor.

Head-to-Knee Pose

Janu Shirshasana (jah-new shear-SHAHS-anna)
janu = knee (compare Latin genu, "knee"); shirsha = head

In the full version of this pose, the hands grip the sides of the extended-leg foot. Here we'll use a strap to work into the forward bend. If you then have the flexibility, you can grip the feet.

1 Sit on a folded blanket in Staff Pose. Place your yoga block face down outside your left leg. Bend your left knee and, with an exhale, draw your heel in toward your perineum.

2 Rest your left knee on the yoga block. *Note: Keep the left shin perpendicular to the right leg while making sure your left sole doesn't slide underneath your right thigh.*

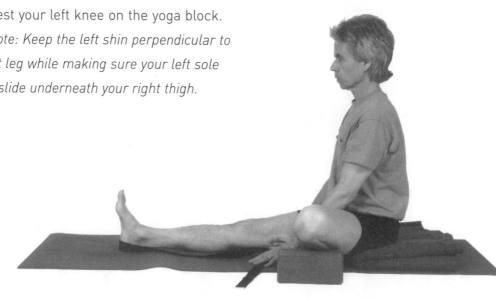

BENEFITS

Head-to-Knee stretches the spine, shoulders, and hamstrings.

CAUTIONS

Avoid this pose if you have a serious back or knee injury.

CHALLENGE YOURSELF

You can increase the challenge in this pose by drawing the bent leg back past the perpendicular—that is, by widening the angle between the two legs past 90 degrees.

3 Wrap the strap around your right sole and walk your hands along the strap toward your right foot until your arms are fully extended. *Note: Make sure your torso is relatively perpendicular to the floor.*

4 Inhale, lift your chest, and, with an exhale, *lightly* walk your hands a few inches along the strap. Inhale, lift your chest again, and, walk your hands a few more inches forward. Continue in this manner until you feel a comfortable stretch in the back of your right leg and your back torso. Then hold for 1 to 3 minutes. *Note: Keep your arms straight (don't bend your elbows), and be sure not to forcefully pull yourself forward into the pose.*

To Come Up: Come up with an inhale.

Seated Wide-Leg Pose

Upavishta Konasana (oo-pah-VEESH-tah cone-AHS-anna)
upavishta = seated, sitting; kona = angle

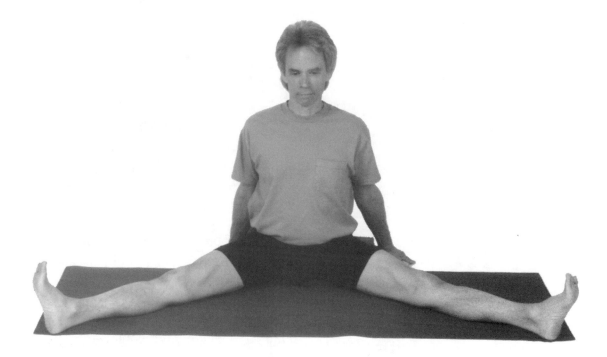

1 From Staff Pose, place your hands on the floor behind your pelvis, lean your torso slightly back, and slide your legs apart. Press through your heels and stretch your soles. *Note: The legs should make an angle of anywhere from 90 to 135 degrees.*

BENEFITS

Seated Wide-Leg stretches the insides and backs of the legs, and strengthens the thighs.

CAUTIONS

Avoid this pose if you have a serious back or groin injury.

CHALLENGE YOURSELF

From step 2, twist your torso to the right. You can use a looped strap, gripped in your left hand, to hold your right foot. Hold for 30 seconds, release with an exhale, then turn for the same length of time to the left.

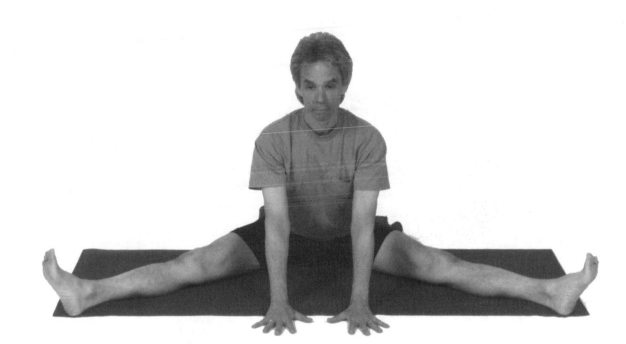

2 Lay your hands on the floor between your legs. Hold for 1 to 3 minutes. *Note: Most beginners will feel a stretch in the backs of the legs with the torso fairly upright. If possible, though, exhale and walk your hands slowly forward until you feel a comfortable stretch in the backs of your legs. As you lean your torso forward, try to keep your knee caps pointing toward the ceiling; press your outer thighs firmly to the floor.*

To Come Up: Come up with an inhale. Bend your knees slightly and, with your hands, scoop your legs together.

Intense Stretch-of-the-West

Paschimottanasana (posh-ee-moh-tan-AHS-anna)
paschimottana = intense stretch of the West (pashima = west; uttana = intense stretch)

In the full version of this pose, the hands grip the outer sides of the feet. Here we'll use a strap to work into the forward bend.

1 Sit on a folded blanket in Staff Pose and wrap the strap around your soles. Walk your hands along the strap toward your feet until your arms are fully extended. *Note: At this point, keep your torso perpendicular to the floor. Press actively through your heels and the bases of your big toes.*

2 Inhale, lift your chest, and with an exhale, *lightly* walk your hands a few inches down the strap. *Note: Keep your arms straight (don't bend your elbows), and be sure not to forcefully pull yourself forward into the pose.*

Intense Stretch-of-the-West Pose stretches the spine, shoulders, hamstrings. Traditional texts say that it also increases your appetite, reduces obesity, and cures diseases.

CAUTION

Avoid this pose if you have a serious back injury.

CHALLENGE YOURSELF

If your flexibility allows, release the strap and grip the outer sides of your feet. To increase the challenge, bend your elbows out to the sides and lightly draw your torso further forward.

3 Inhale, lift your chest again, and walk your hands a few more inches forward. Continue in this manner until you feel a comfortable stretch in the backs of your legs and your back torso. Hold for 1 to 3 minutes. *Note: Periodically, with an inhalation, lift and lengthen your front torso, then lower down again on the exhalation.*

To Come Up: Inhale back to Staff Pose.

sitting twists

Sitting twists have similar benefits and cautions. First, they all "squeeze and soak" the intervertebral disks, the (relatively) round, spongy pads that separate the spinal vertebrae; the principle is much like squeezing and soaking a sponge. The twisting movement itself squeezes the disk, wringing out all the "dirty water"; then when you release the twist, "clean water"—spinal fluids and blood—is soaked up. This keeps the disks supple well into old age.

The twists also stretch the hips and chest, massage the belly and the belly organs, and help release lower back tension. But if you have a serious lower back injury, especially a bulging intervertebral disk, you should avoid these poses unless you're practicing with the supervision of an experienced teacher.

TIPS

Just as in the sitting forward bends, beginners need to sit on a blanket support for the sitting twists. It's absolutely essential that you begin these twists with a neutral pelvis and a long (although not straight) spine. In the first pose, the blanket should be wedged only under the buttock you're twisting toward. In the other two poses, both buttocks should sit evenly on the blanket.

There are two ways to twist your neck and head in these poses. You can turn your neck and head in the direction of the twist; when you're twisting to the right (for example), you'll turn your head to look over your right shoulder. Alternatively, you can turn your neck and head to oppose the twist of the torso; that means looking over your left shoulder during a right twist.

All the poses in this section begin and end in Staff Pose (see page 74).

PROPS: For the twists, you'll need a blanket and, optionally, a strap.

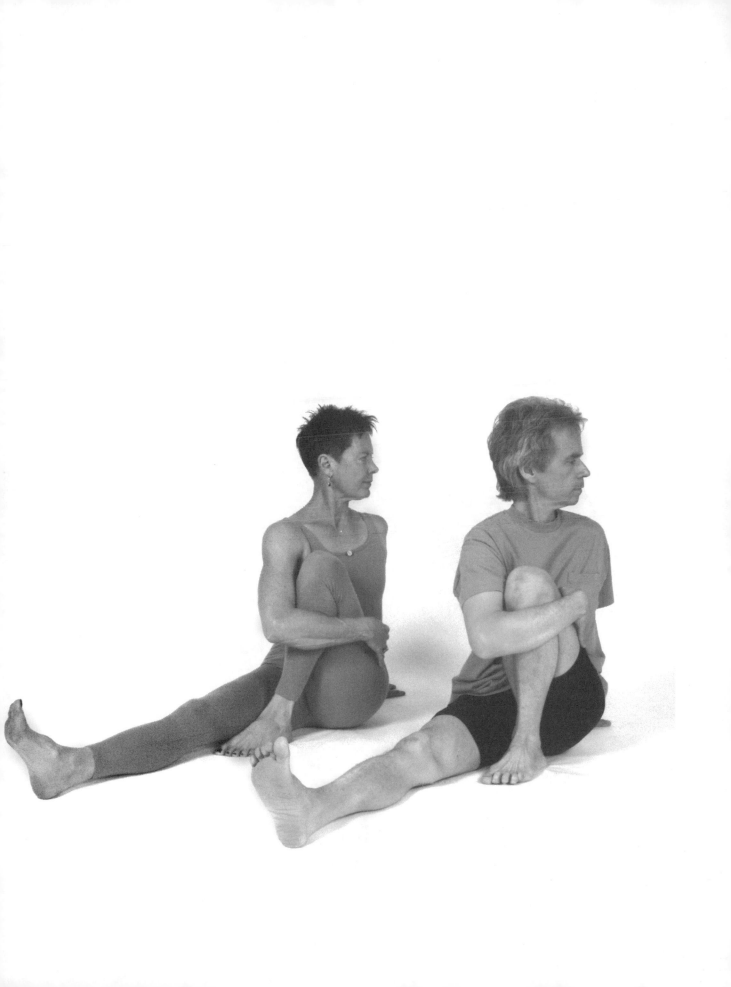

Bharadvaja's Pose

Perform to the right then repeat to the left

Bharadvajasana (bah-rod-va-JAHS-anna)
Bharadvaja = literally means both "skylark" and "bearing" (i.e., the speed or strength of flight). Bharadvaja is a legendary Hindu sage.

The pose described here is a modified version of the full pose. In the full pose, the hand that's pressed to the floor here is instead wrapped around the back torso to grip the opposite arm above the elbow.

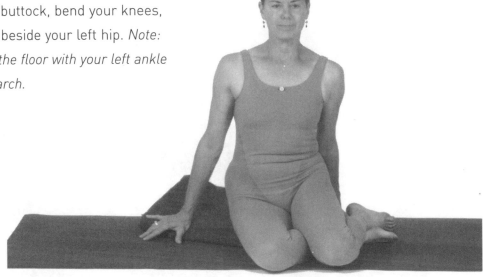

1 Sit on a folded blanket in Staff Pose. Shift onto your right buttock, bend your knees, and pull your feet in beside your left hip. *Note: Position your feet on the floor with your left ankle nestled in your right arch.*

2 Exhale and twist your torso to the right. Clasp your right knee with your left hand and press your right fingertips firmly against the floor beside your right buttock. *Note: Keep your left buttock close to the floor by pressing your left thigh toward the floor.*

CHALLENGE YOURSELF

Here's a way to increase the twist. In this example, you'll be twisting to your right. Hold the strap doubled over (in a large loop) in your right hand. Perform the twist, then exhale and sweep your right arm and the loop around behind your back torso, parallel to your waist. Slip your left arm through the loop, and slide the loop up to just above the elbow. Walk your right hand along the strap as close as possible to the left arm. Lean back slightly against the forearm to increase the twist. Then reverse the arms when twisting to your left.

3 On each inhale, the spine naturally lengthens. With every exhale, see if you can twist a little more. Hold for 30 seconds to 1 minute. *Note: Make sure that your belly stays soft.*

To Come Up: Release with an exhale and return to Staff.

Marichi's Pose

Marichyasana (mar-ee-chee-AHS-anna)
Marichi = literally means "a ray of light" (of the sun or moon). Marichi is a legendary Hindu sage.

The pose described here is a modified version of the full pose.

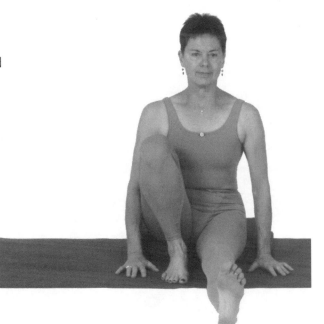

1 Sit on a folded blanket in Staff Pose. Bend your right knee and set your foot on the floor, your heel just in front of your buttock. *Note: Press your inner right foot firmly to the floor. Keep your left leg active by extending through your heel.*

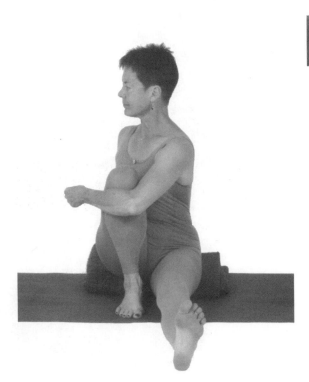

2 Exhale and turn to the right. Hug your right leg with your left arm, and press your right fingertips against the floor, behind and to the outside of the right hip. *Note: Push your right fingertips against the floor to move your torso up and forward, closing your left side against your right thigh.*

If you find your torso tipping back
away from the bent leg, even though
you're sitting on a blanket, perform
the pose about 18 to 24 inches away
from a wall, with the wall to your back
torso when facing your legs. When
you twist, press your free hand against
the wall and push your torso forward.

CHALLENGE YOURSELF

Try the full version of this pose by
bringing the opposite arm to the
outside of the bent-knee leg then
wrapping it back around the leg. The
free arm is next wrapped behind the
back, and its hand used to grip the
opposite wrist.

3 With each inhale, lift your navel up, along
the inside of your right side, and lengthen
your spine. Then with each exhale, twist to the
right a little bit more. Hold for 30 seconds to 1
minute.

To Come Up: Release
with an exhale and
return to Staff.

Lord-of-the-Fishes Pose

Also called the Half Lord-of-the-Fishes Pose

Matsyendrasana (mot-see-en-DRAHS-anna)

Matsyendra = king of the fish (matsya = fish; indra = ruler), a legendary teacher of Yoga

The pose described here is a modified version of the full pose, in which the arms and hands are used very much as described for Marichi's Pose.

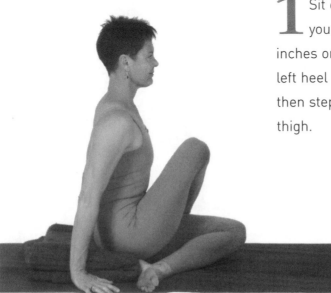

1 Sit on a folded blanket in Staff Pose. Bend your knees and set your feet on the floor, 12 inches or so away from your buttocks. Slide your left heel beneath the outside of your right hip, then step your right foot to the outside of your left thigh.

2 Exhale and turn to the right. Hug your right leg with your left arm, and press your right fingertips against the floor, behind and to the outside of the right hip. *Note: Push your right fingertips against the floor to move your torso up and forward, closing your left side against your right thigh.*

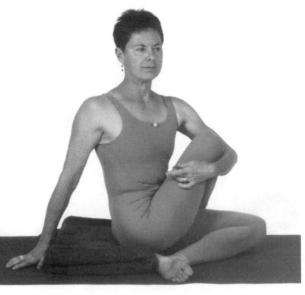

CAUTIONS

Avoid this exercise if you have any shoulder or neck injuries.

TIPS

This twist is often hindered by tightness in the outer hip of the bent-knee leg. Burrow the thumb of your free hand deeply into the bent-knee groin. Then, softening the groin, press the outer hip firmly down toward the floor.

For best results with this exercise, be sure to keep your elbows as straight as possible as you make the circles. Also keep your arms equidistant from your head; don't let them angle off to one side or the other.

3 With each inhale, lift your navel up, along the inside of your right side, and lengthen your spine. Then with each exhale, twist to the right a little bit more. Hold for 30 seconds to 1 minute.

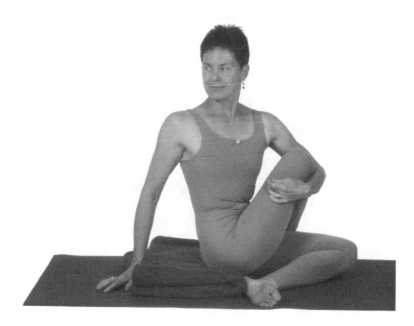

To Come Up: Release with an exhale and return to Staff.

back bends

Most of your daily movements involve bending forward or twisting to the sides. You're unlikely to bend over backward—literally or figuratively. As a result, the front of your torso has become shortened and you're hunched over.

Back bends help to remedy this situation by stretching the front body, specifically the thighs and front groins, belly, chest, and shoulders, and the deep hip flexors (the psoas pair; see page 58). This generally helps to improve posture. Back bends also strengthen the backs of the legs, the buttocks, and the muscles that run along the sides of the spine. But all of these poses should be avoided if you have any serious back, shoulder, or neck injuries, or if you have high blood pressure.

Additionally, two of the poses, Intense Stretch-of-the-East and Upward Facing Dog, strengthen the wrists and arms, although these poses should be avoided if you have serious wrist injuries.

TIPS

In the prone poses (Locust, Bow, and Cobra) and the kneeling pose (Camel), you can pad the floor with a folded blanket.

PROPS: For the back bends, you'll need a chair, a strap, and a blanket.

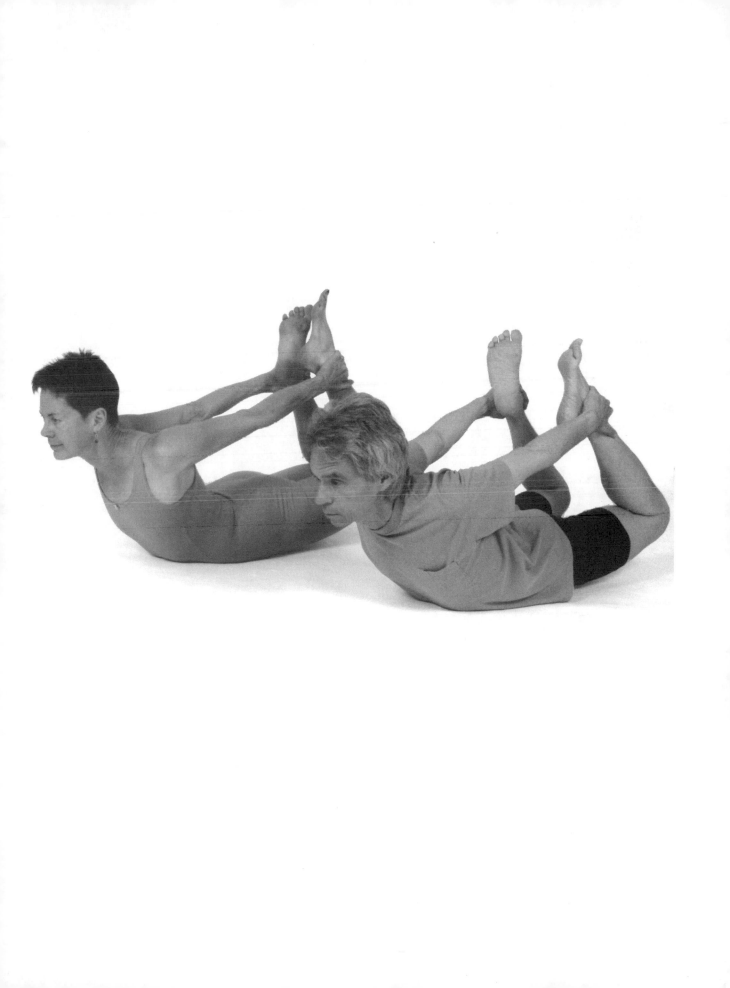

Locust Pose

Shalabhasana (sha-lah-BAHS-anna)
shalabha = locust, grasshopper

As your practice of the asanas progresses, you may run across a few variations of this simple back bend. One of them is described in the Tips.

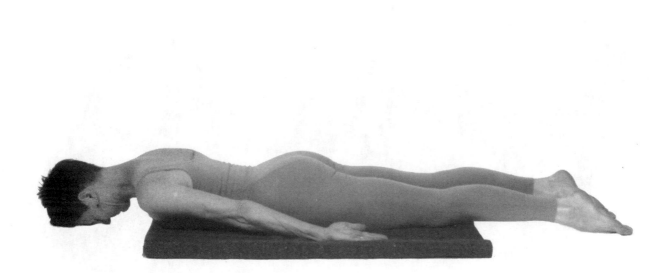

1 Lie face down with your body resting on a folded blanket, arms stretched alongside your torso, palms up, forehead resting on the floor. *Note: Press your tail slightly down, toward your pubis.*

Back bends stretch the front body, specifically the thighs and groins, belly, chest, shoulders, and the deep hip flexors (the psoas pair); this generally helps to improve posture. Back bends also strengthen the backs of the legs, the buttocks, and the muscles that run along the sides of the spine.

CAUTIONS

Avoid all back bends if you have a serious back injury, shoulder or neck injury, or high blood pressure.

TIPS

Be sure to keep your thighs rotated slightly inward.

If you have difficulty holding your raised legs in place, support them on a block.

CHALLENGE YOURSELF

You can also perform this pose with your hands clasped behind your head. This pose is called the Sea Monster (Makarasana, pronounced mah-KAH-rahs-anna, which is also rendered as "crocodile" or "dolphin").

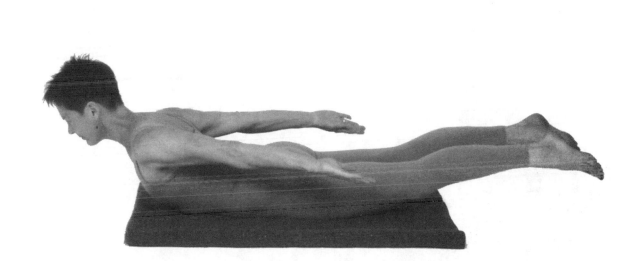

2 Inhale and simultaneously lift your head, upper torso, arms, and legs away from the floor. Look straight ahead. Raise your legs until the tops of your thighs just clear the floor, and raise your arms approximately parallel to the floor. Reach actively back through your toetips and fingertips. Hold for 30 seconds to 1 minute. *Note: Firm (but don't harden) your buttocks to raise your legs; keep your pubis, hip points, belly, and lower ribs pressed to the floor.*

To Come Up: Release back to the floor with an exhale.

Intense Stretch-of-the-East

Repeat this pose 2 or 3 times.

Purvottanasana (poor-voh-tahn-AHS-anna)
purvottana = intense stretch of the East (purva = east; uttana = intense stretch)

In Hatha Yoga, the front of the body is thought of as the East, the back of the body the West (paschima).
The full pose is performed with your hands and feet on the floor; here, though, we'll use a chair, positioned a
few inches away from a wall, to support the head.

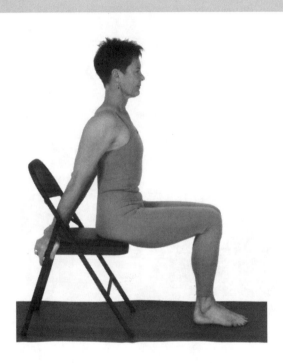

1 Place a chair with its back a couple of inches away from a wall. Sit on the front edge of your chair seat, knees bent at right angles, feet on the floor. Grip the back edge of the chair seat with your hands. *Note: Your thumbs should be pointing away from each other.*

2 Inhale, push your feet against the floor and your hands against the chair seat, and lift your pelvis up until you make one long, diagonal line from your knees to your shoulders. Lay your head lightly back against the wall. *Note: Your shins should be relatively perpendicular to the floor.*

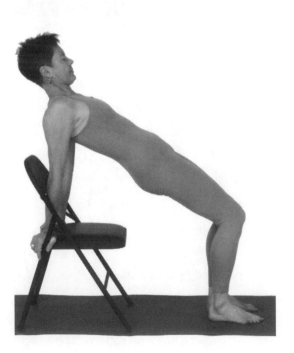

CHALLENGE YOURSELF

When you feel that you've sufficient strength, perform this pose as described above, but without the chair. Sit on the floor with your hands slightly behind your pelvis, fingers pointing forward, knees bent, feet on the floor. Inhale and lift your pelvis up until your torso and thighs are relatively parallel to the floor, shins and arms perpendicular. Then inhale each leg straight, holding your torso parallel to the floor.

3 Pressing your tail toward the ceiling, inhale and stretch your right leg out straight. *Note: Once extended, firm the inner foot against the floor.*

4 Then stretch your left leg out straight. Hold for 30 seconds to 1 minute. *Note: Your feet should be slightly pigeon-toed when extended.*

To Come Up: Release your buttocks back to the chair seat with an exhale.

103

Bow Pose

Dhanurasana (don-your-AHS-anna)
dhanu = bow

Repeat this pose 2 or 3 times.

When you look at this pose from the side, you'll see that the torso and legs make the body of the bow, and the arms the bowstring.

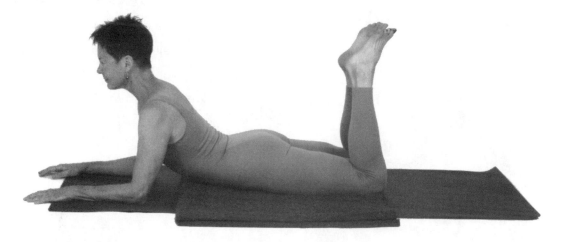

1 Lie face down on a folded blanket supporting you from your knees to above your hips. Exhale, bend your knees, and draw your heels toward your buttocks.

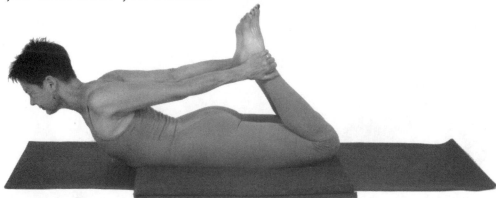

2 With another exhale, reach back with your hands and grip your ankles. *Note: Be sure to grasp your ankles, not the tops of your feet. Keep your thighs parallel—don't allow them to splay wider than your hips.*

TIP

If you find it difficult to grip your ankles directly, hold a strap in your hands and wrap it around your ankles.

CHALLENGE YOURSELF

Perform the pose as described above. Then with an exhale, slowly roll over onto your right side. Hold there for a few seconds, looking upward toward the ceiling. Exhale, roll back onto your belly, then exhale again and roll to your left. Again hold for a few seconds, and finally roll back to your belly with an exhale. This pose is called Side Bow (parshva dhanurasana).

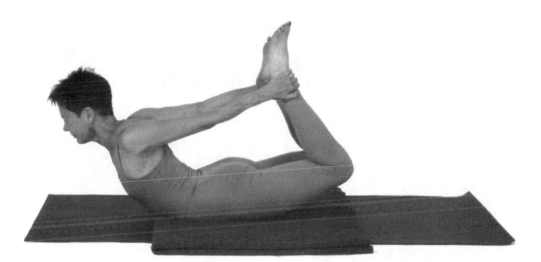

3 Inhale and slowly lift your heels up and away from your buttocks. As you do so, your upper torso will lift away from the floor. Firm your buttocks and press your tail toward your pubis. Look straight ahead. Hold for 30 seconds to 1 minute. *Note: You can keep your thighs on the floor, or lift them a few inches off the floor. In either case, continue to press your pubis firmly to the floor.*

To Come Up: Release back to the floor with an exhale.

Serpent Pose

Commonly called the Cobra Pose

Bhujangasana (boo-jang-GAHS-anna)

bhujanga = serpent, snake. In Sanskrit, bhuj *means "bend, curved,"* anga *"limb"; so* bhujanga *literally means "crooked limb."* Bhuj *is the etymological root of the English word "bow."*

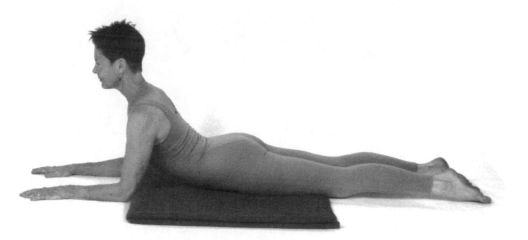

1 Lie on a folded blanket with your arms extended out past your head and spread your palms on the floor. *Note: Firm your buttocks and press your tail downward and lift your navel away from your pubis.*

2 As you bend your elbows, slide your forearms back toward your torso and lift your upper torso and head away from the floor. Look straight ahead. *Note: Position your elbows under your shoulders (upper arms are perpendicular to the floor) and make sure that your forearms are parallel to each other. Draw your shoulders down, away from your ears, and lift your chest.*

CAUTION

As you straighten and lift your elbows, be careful not to crunch your lower back. Keep your elbows slightly bent if necessary.

TIPS

If you want to straighten your elbows but also want to protect your lower back, slide your hands forward a few inches.

When you lift your torso, think of moving it up and *forward*, not up and back. This will protect your lower back.

CHALLENGE YOURSELF

Once you've lifted into the full pose as described above, you can increase the stretch of the front torso by walking your hands back below your shoulders (so the arms are perpendicular to the floor).

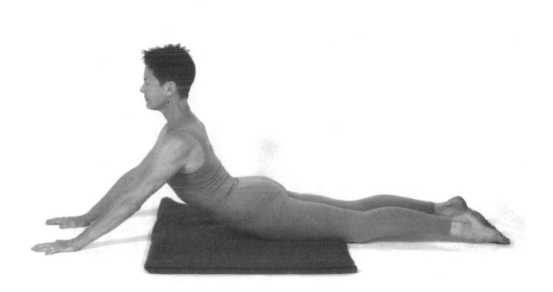

3 Slowly straighten and lift your elbows away from the floor. Hold for 30 seconds to 1 minute.

To Come Up: Release with an exhale.

Camel Pose

Ustrasana (oosh-TRAHS-anna)
ustra = camel

In the full pose, your hands are pressed against your soles. Here we'll use a chair to support your hands.

1 Kneel on a folded blanket, knees slightly apart, thighs perpendicular to the floor. Set your chair behind you, with the front edge of the seat lightly touching your buttocks. *Note: Actively press your shins and the tops of your feet firmly against the floor.*

2 Spread your palms on the back of your pelvis, fingers pointing down. Press your upper buttocks down, toward your tail bone, and then lengthen through your tail bone to the floor. *Note: Prevent your front groins from bowing out; hold your front thighs back, resisting the downward movement of the tail bone.*

TIP

Once in position, widen your scapulae across your back.

CHALLENGE YOURSELF

You can increase the challenge of Camel by performing the full pose, with your palms pressing against your soles, either with your toes turned under and your heels elevated, or with the tops of your feet on the floor.

3 Lean back against the resistance of your hands, and lift your chest toward the ceiling. Carefully release your hands and grip the sides of the chair seat. *Note: Be sure not to collapse onto your lower back or squeeze the back of your neck by dropping your head too far back.*

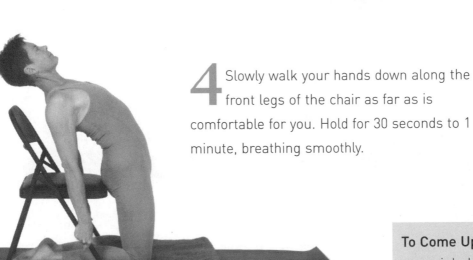

4 Slowly walk your hands down along the front legs of the chair as far as is comfortable for you. Hold for 30 seconds to 1 minute, breathing smoothly.

To Come Up: Come up on an inhale, leading with your chest, letting your head follow.

Upward Facing Dog Pose

Urdhva Mukha Shvanasana (erd-vah moo-kah shvon-AHS-anna)
urdhva mukha = face upward (urdhva = upward; mukha = face); shvana = dog

Upward Facing Dog Pose is similar to Serpent, except that the legs and pelvis are lifted off the floor, and the hands are positioned below the shoulder so the arms are perpendicular to the floor.

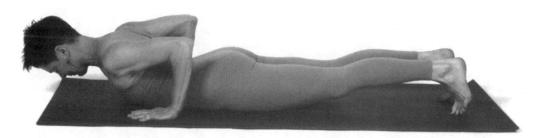

1 Lie on your belly with your toes turned under. Set your hands on the floor beside your waist so that your forearms are perpendicular to the floor.

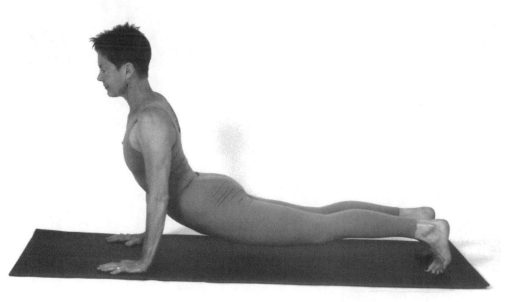

2 Inhale, press your hands and toes against the floor, and slowly straighten your arms. As you do so, simultaneously lift your legs and pelvis off the floor. *Note: Be sure to firm (but don't harden) your buttocks, and press your tail toward your pubis.*

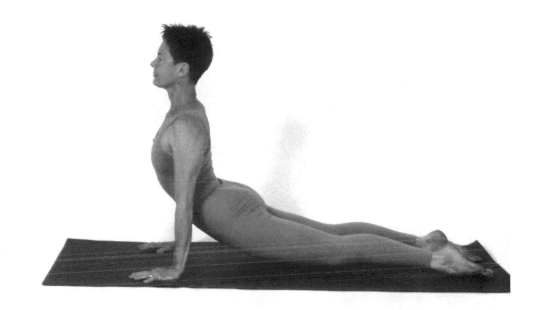

3 Arch your torso up and through your arms. Look straight ahead. Hold for 30
seconds to 1 minute. *Note: If you prefer, you can tip your head slightly back and gaze
toward the ceiling. In either case, make sure to draw your shoulders down away from your
ears.*

To Come Up: Release
with an exhale back to
the support.

shoulder stand and plow

Shoulder Stand (or All-Limb Pose) is often called the queen of the asanas. It and the Plow, when done properly, afford a wonderful stretch to the neck and shoulders. When done improperly, however, they can cause a good deal of damage to the neck and shoulders.

Shoulder Stand and Plow are often pictured with the practitioner's shoulders flat on the floor, or maybe lifted slightly above the floor on a single folded blanket. Be aware that this is an advanced version of the pose, requiring open shoulders and a tension-free neck. A beginning student, however, usually has tight shoulders and a tense, shortened neck. Until you are experienced, never perform Shoulder Stand or Plow without a several-inches-thick blanket support for your shoulders and upper arms. This support will protect your neck from strain and possible serious injury. You'll also use this support for the first pose in this section, Bridge Pose, which is a preparation for Shoulder Stand.

To make a Shoulder Stand support, you'll need at least three firm blankets. Fold each blanket into a rectangle measuring about 18 x 30 inches. Then look at the two 30-inch sides of each blanket: there's a firm side (where the blanket's folded over), and an open side. Stack the blankets so that the firm sides are one atop another. If you find, once you're on this support, that your neck still feels strained, then add one or more blankets until your back neck is long and your throat is soft.

TIPS

For Shoulder Stand and Plow, set your stack of blankets about a foot or so away from your yoga wall, with the 30-inch firm sides farthest from the wall. In these two poses, tightness in your shoulders can cause your elbows to slide apart; this, in turn, can collapse your torso onto your upper back, straining your neck and making a challenging position even more challenging. Fold a sticky mat in half and lay it over the bottom half of the blanket (the half closer to the wall, where your elbows will be), or roll the mat up and lay it near the open sides of the blankets (again, to support your elbows).

PROPS: You'll need at least three blankets, a strap, and one or possibly two sticky mats. For Modified Shoulder Stand, you'll also need a chair.

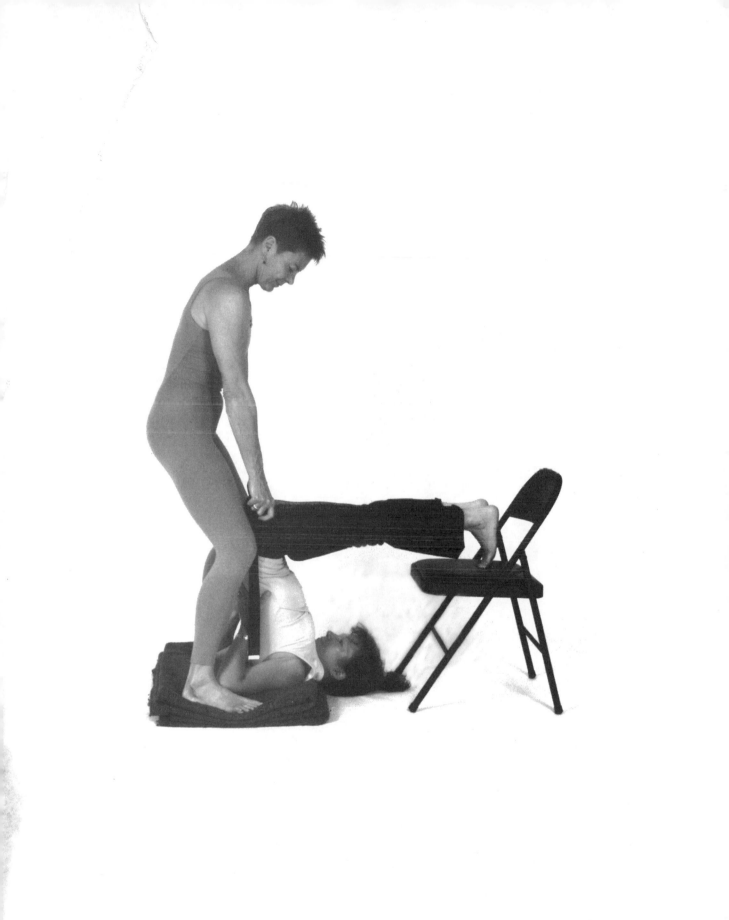

Bridge Pose

Setu Bandha (set-too BAHN-dah)
setu = dam, dike, or bridge; bandha = construction

Repeat 2 or 3 times, each time trying to lift your pelvis a little higher

Bridge Pose is technically a back bend, but it's also an excellent preparation for Shoulder Stand and Plow. In the full pose, the hands clasp the ankles; here we'll use a strap to secure your hands to your ankles.

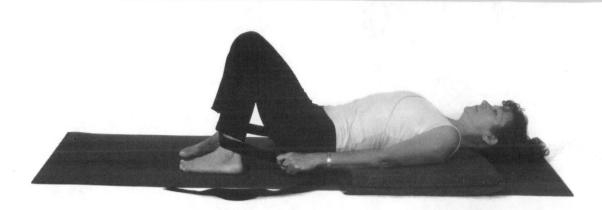

1 Lie on your back with your shoulders supported on your blanket stack. Bend your knees and swing the strap over your knees and draw it down around your ankles. Walk your hands along the strap until your arms are straight. *Note: Make sure your feet are flat on the floor, heels close to your buttocks and toes slightly pigeon-toed.*

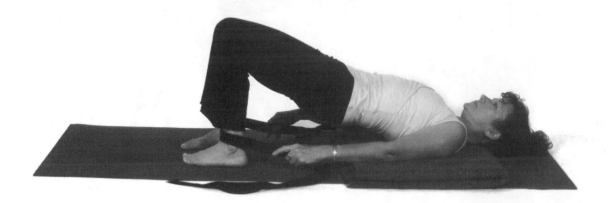

2 Press your inner feet and the backs of your arms against the floor, and lift your pelvis with an inhale. *Note: Firm (but don't harden) your buttocks, pressing your tail toward your pubis. Be sure to keep your thighs parallel; don't let your knees splay outward.*

BENEFITS

Bridge stretches the front of the thighs, the belly and chest, the shoulders, and the back of the neck.

CAUTIONS

Avoid this pose if you have a serious neck, knee, or lower back injury.

TIP

Squeeze a block between your thighs if you have difficulty keeping them parallel while in this pose.

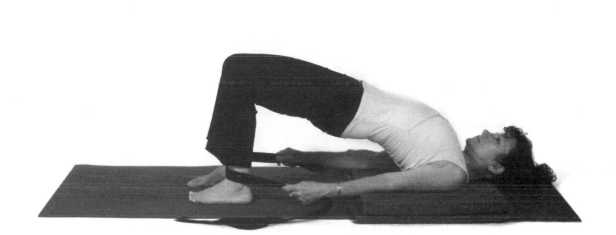

3 Continue lifting your pelvis until you create a smooth diagonal line from your knees to the top of your sternum. Hold for 1 or 2 minutes. *Note: Lift your chin slightly away from your chest. Broaden, don't squeeze, your shoulder blades.*

To Come Up: Release with an exhale.

All-Limb Pose

Commonly called Shoulder Stand
Sarvangasana (sar-vang-GAHS-anna)
sarva = all; anga = limb

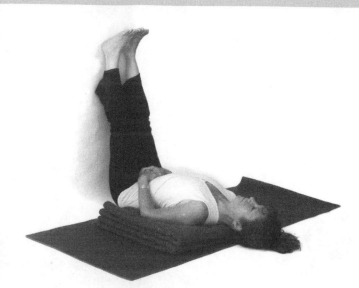

1 Lie on your blanket stack with your legs up the wall, elbows alongside your torso on the blankets. *Note: Your shoulders should be a couple of inches in from the fold side of the blankets; your head should be on the floor.*

2 Bend your knees, press your feet against the wall, and with an inhale, lift your pelvis away from the blankets until it's over your shoulders, perpendicular to the floor. Bending at the elbow, steady your torso with your hands. *Note: For your hands to provide good support, press the back of your upper arms against the blanket stack and spread your palms against your back as high up as possible. Your elbows should be slightly wider than your shoulders.*

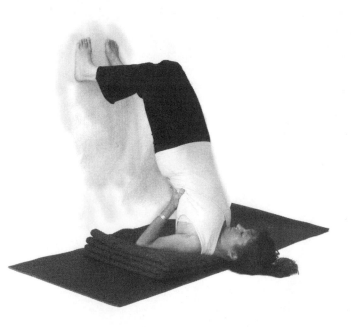

BENEFITS

Shoulder Stand is considered to be a "neutralizing" pose: it will quiet an overly stimulated brain, and stimulate a dull one. It also stretches the shoulders, chest, and neck.

CAUTIONS

DO NOT perform Sarvangasana if you have high blood pressure, if you're menstruating or more than 3 months pregnant, or if you have a neck injury. Once you're in Sarvangasana, DO NOT turn your head to look to the side. ALWAYS look straight up at the tips of your toes.

TIPS

In Shoulder Stand, be sure to press through the bases of your big toes and inner heels toward the ceiling (the same pressure you'd apply if you were standing on the floor). Imagine that your inner legs are slightly longer than your outer legs.

3 Now straighten your knees, one at a time, and extend through your heels toward the ceiling. *Note: If you find yourself in the Banana-asana (see photo), firm your buttocks, bring your tail slightly forward (toward your pubis), and stretch your legs back so that the tips of your toes line up over your eyes.*

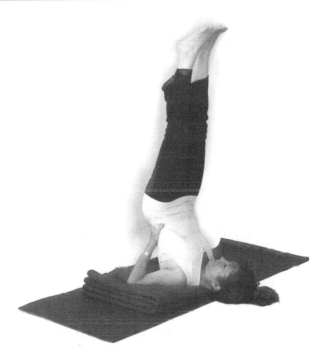

4 At first, hold for about 30 seconds. Slowly add 5 to 10 seconds until you reach 3 minutes. Continue for 3 minutes each practice for another week, then repeat the above process, gradually adding a few seconds every time until you can comfortably hold the pose for 5 minutes. *Note: You should lift your chin slightly away from your sternum to soften your throat.*

To Come Down: Bend your knees, lightly touch your feet to the wall, and release your torso with an exhale to the support.

Plow Pose

Halasana (hah-LAHS-anna)
hala = plow

In the full Plow, the toes rest on the floor, but in this book we'll rest the toes on a chair support.

1 Perform Shoulder Stand (All-Limb Pose) as previously described but with a chair 18 to 24 inches (depending on your height) behind your blankets. *Note: Remember to hold your torso perpendicular to the floor as much as you can during this entire pose.*

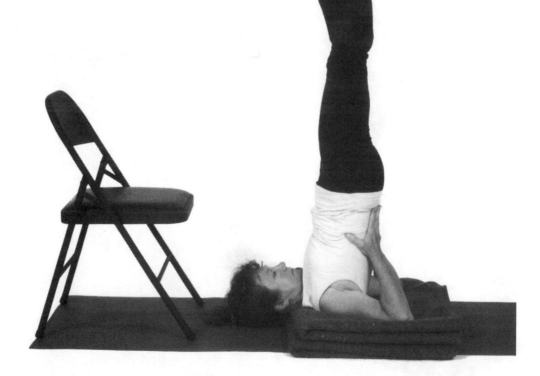

BENEFITS

Plow is considered to be a "neutralizing" pose: it will quiet an overly stimulated brain, and stimulate a dull one. It also stretches the shoulders, chest, and neck.

CAUTIONS

DO NOT perform Halasana if you have high blood pressure, if you're menstruating or more than 3 months pregnant, or if you have a neck injury.

Once you're in Halasana, DO NOT turn your head to look to the side. ALWAYS look straight up at the tips of your toes.

TIP

Many beginners find it difficult (if not impossible) to lift out of Plow with their legs together. To improve your chances, lean your pelvis back slightly (away from the chair) and draw your inner groins deep into your pelvis to initiate the movement.

CHALLENGE YOURSELF

After lowering your feet to the chair, try removing your hand support of the torso. Reach your hands out onto the floor behind your back, press your arms firmly to the floor, and clasp your hands.

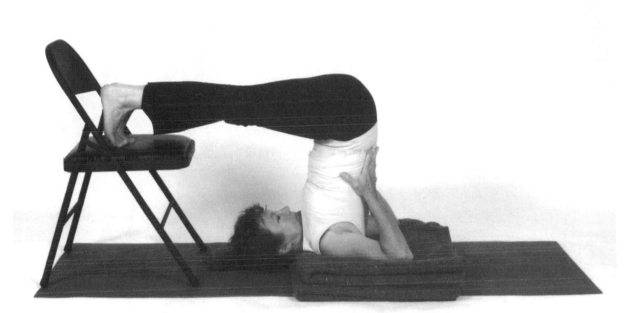

2 Exhale and slowly lower your feet to the chair seat. Start by holding for 15 seconds, and gradually work your way up to 1 to 2 minutes. *Note: Keep your knees fully extended by pressing actively through your heels toward the chair back, and (without lifting your feet away from the chair seat) press your thighs toward the ceiling.*

To Come Out: Press your hands against your back torso, inhale, and try to lift your legs back to vertical simultaneously (not one at a time). From Shoulder Stand, bend your knees, touch your feet to the wall, and release your torso with an exhale to the support.

Modified Shoulder Stand

Modified Shoulder Stand is performed with the support of a chair. It's a pose midway between the full, active version in this section and the passive Inverted Action Pose (page 124).

1 Fold your sticky mat up four times and lay it across the front edge of your chair seat. Fold two blankets into 10 x 30-inch rectangles and stack them a few inches away from the chair legs, with the firm sides facing away from the chair. Straddle the chair seat, facing the chair back, then swing your legs over the chair back, hooking your knees on the top edge of the back. Grip the sides of the chair back or the legs just below the back.

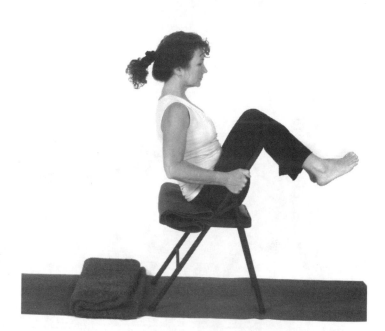

2 Exhale, lean back, and slowly lower your shoulders lightly onto the blankets. *Note: Make sure the firm edges of the blankets are right below the line of your shoulders. The back of your pelvis should rest on the front edge of the seat, padded by the sticky mat.*

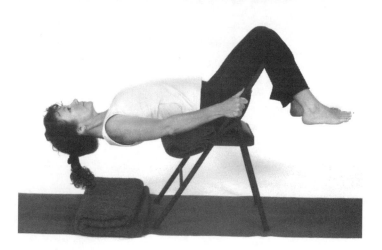

BENEFITS

Modified Shoulder Stand is considered to be a "neutralizing" pose: it will quiet an overly stimulated brain, and stimulate a dull one. It also stretches the shoulders, chest, and neck.

CAUTIONS

Be sure to keep your neck long, but at the same time don't overstretch it. Lift the tops of your shoulders slightly *toward* your ears. If necessary, add another blanket to your stack. DO NOT perform Modified Shoulder Stand if you have high blood pressure, if you're menstruating or more than 3 months pregnant, or if you have a neck injury. Once you're in Modified Shoulder Stand, DO NOT turn your head to look to the side. ALWAYS look straight up at the tips of your toes.

TIP

Taller people should roll up the sticky mat to provide extra height below their pelvis.

3 Slip your arms underneath the seat, over the front rung, between the front legs (if you're tighter in the shoulders, reach outside the legs), and grip the back legs or rung of the chair.

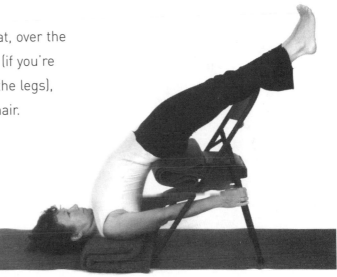

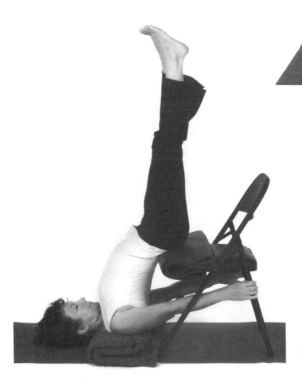

4 Inhale and extend your legs perpendicular to the floor. Hold for 30 seconds. Gradually build up your stay in the pose to about 5 minutes. *Note: Make sure not to lift your buttocks away from the seat.*

To Come Down: Bend your knees and rest your feet on the top edge of the chair back. Release the chair legs, slide the chair away from you, drop your feet to the seat, then push the chair away to lower your torso to the floor.

restoratives

Restoratives are cool-down poses, used either at the end of a practice, or between poses during a practice. The ultimate restorative is Corpse Pose (see page 128).

Although there are only three restoratives in this section, there are a few other poses in parts II and III that can also be used in this way. For example, Twist-around-the-Belly (see page 62) or the forward bend wall-hang (see page 18) might be used as a cool-down after a back bend; Inverted Action Pose (see page 124) can be a nice cool-down after a vigorous practice, a preparation for Corpse, or even a practice-ender in itself.

TIPS

Whenever practicing in cool or cold weather, be sure that you'll be warm during your time in the restorative pose or poses, especially if you tend toward chilliness. Put on your socks and a loose-fitting sweater or sweatshirt, or you can even cover yourself with a blanket or two. Take off your glasses.

PROPS: For restoratives, you might want a bolster or two rolled-up blankets, and an eye bag.

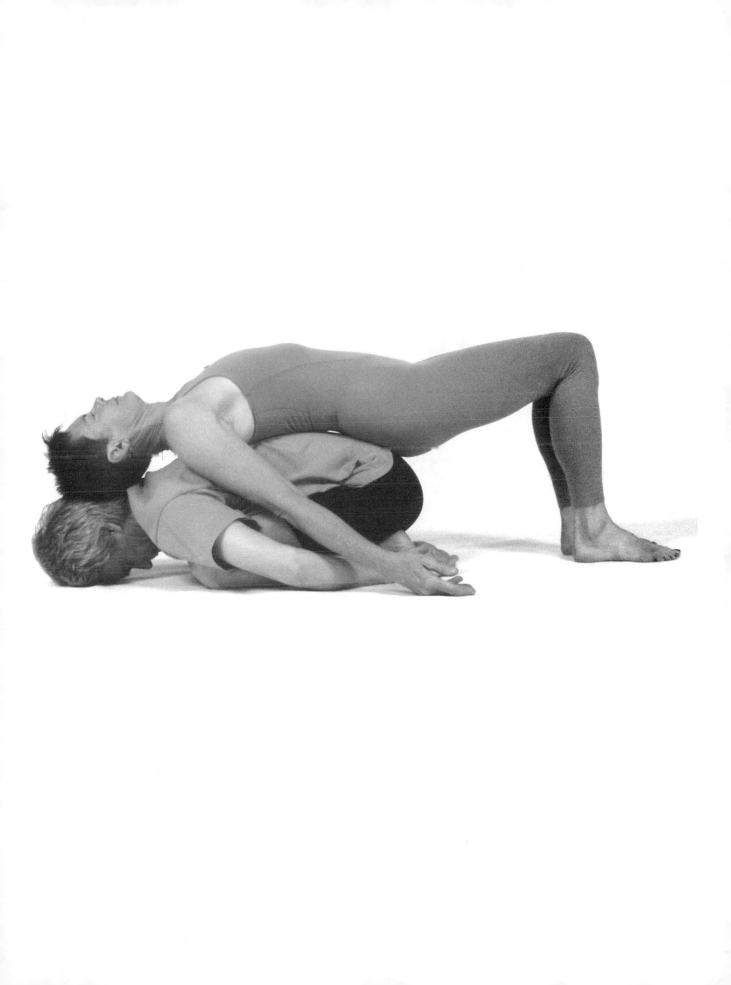

Inverted Action Pose

Viparita karani (vip-par-ee-tah car-AHN-ee)
viparita = turned around, reversed, inverted; karani = doing, making, action

Traditionally, Viparita Karani isn't categorized as an asana; rather, it's called a "seal" (*mudra*), its full name Viparita Karani Mudra. In some old texts, it seems to be performed as a Headstand (*shirshasana*), a pose not included in this book; in others, it's described as Shoulder Stand (*sarvangasana*) (see page 116). Today, Viparita Karani names a pose that's a supported variation of Shoulder Stand.

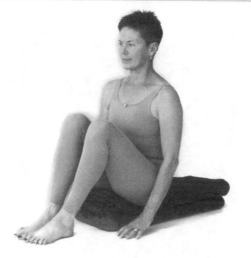

1 Fold blankets into long thick rectangles and stack them one atop the other about 5 or 6 inches away from the wall. Sit sideways on one end of the support with the side of your torso up against the wall, knees bent, feet on the floor.

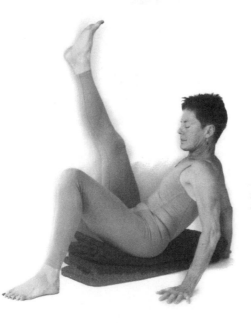

2 Exhale, twist your front torso toward the wall, lean slightly back, and in one smooth movement swing your legs up onto the wall and your shoulders and head down onto the floor.

BENEFITS

Inverted Action soothes tired or cramped legs and feet; gently stretches the back legs, front torso, and the back of the neck; helps relieve a mild backache; and calms the brain.

CAUTIONS

There's some debate about performing this pose during menstruation since it can be considered an inversion; some teachers recommend it, others avoid it. Check with your teacher. Avoid this pose if you have serious eye problems, such as glaucoma, or serious neck or back problems. If your feet start tingling, bend your knees to the sides, touch your soles together, and slide the outer edges of your feet down the wall, bringing your heels close to your pelvis.

TIP

If you have a difficult time holding your legs vertically, secure them with a strap drawn around your thighs just above your knees.

3 With your legs on the wall and shoulders and head resting lightly on the floor, press lightly through your heels toward the ceiling. Stay anywhere from 5 to 15 minutes. *Note: Sink your femur heads deep into your pelvis. Your sitting bones should be slightly away from the wall, "dripping" into the space between the wall and the blankets. Your front torso should create a graceful arch from your pubis to your sternum. If it seems flat or slightly hollow, wiggle your buttocks closer to the wall.*

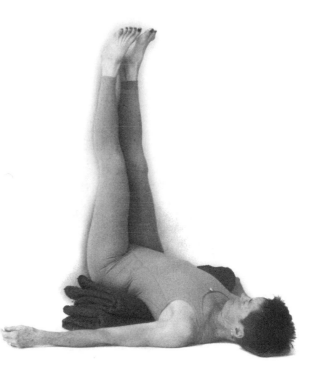

To Come Up: Don't twist off the support. Either slide back until your buttocks are on the floor, or push your feet against the wall, lift your buttocks, slide the support to one side, and lower your torso to the floor.

Child's Pose

Balasana (bah-LAHS-anna)
bala = child

Balasana is a favorite resting pose, either between individual asanas or near the end of an asana practice. It gets its name from its fetal-like shape.

1 Kneel with your big toes touching and your knees hip-width apart. Sit on your heels.

2 With an exhale, fold your torso onto your thighs and lay your forehead on the floor. Rest your hands, palms up, on the floor beside your feet.
Note: Sink the weight of your shoulders and broaden the two sides of your back torso away from your spine. Then lift the base of your skull slightly away from the back of your neck and lengthen your tail out onto the floor behind your pelvis.

Child's Pose gently stretches the front ankles, the thighs, and the back torso. It also quiets the brain and relieves stress.

With a knee injury, perform this pose with a folded blanket wedged between your thighs and calves; if the injury is serious, avoid this pose. Instead, sit cross-legged on the floor and rest your crossed arms and forehead on the front edge of a chair seat.

There's a kind of inverted variation of Child's Pose called the Wind-Freeing Pose (Pavana Muktasana, pronounced pah-vah-nah-mook-TAHS-anna). Lie on your back and, with an exhale, bend your knees and draw your thighs into your belly. Wrap your arms around your shins and squeeze your thighs against your belly. Rock gently from side to side, spreading your back against the floor.

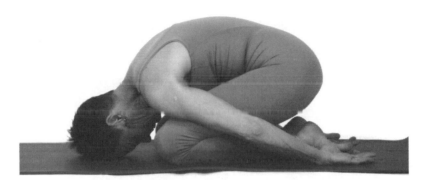

3 Round your back torso like a dome. With each inhale, expand this dome toward the ceiling; with each exhale, nestle your torso more deeply into your thighs. Stay in this pose anywhere from 1 to 3 minutes.

To Come Up: First lengthen the front of your torso, then lift slowly with a smooth inhale.

Corpse Pose

Shavasana (shah-VAHS-anna)
shava = corpse

Yes, Corpse *is* kind of a daunting name for a yoga asana, and many newcomers to the practice tend to avoid this pose or give it short shrift. After all, what's so important about lying on the floor and—typically at first—snoring? Believe me, Corpse is one of the most useful of the poses, one you'll eventually want to practice everyday, regardless of what else you've done.

Actually, Corpse is a lot more complicated than it seems at first glance. Just like any of the other poses, it requires physical alignment. Most beginners, when they recline on the floor, are more or less out of alignment—in the legs and arms, torso, head, the list goes on and on. But this misalignment, whatever it consists of, feels "natural"and so very difficult to self-correct. I often re-arrange students in Corpse, and a standard response is: "Are you *sure* I'm straight?"

You might ask a yoga friend to check your habitual Corpse. Have her look especially at your:

- *Heels*. Both of your heels should be resting on the same spot; frequently the feet are angled slightly differently.
- *Pelvis*. Look at your two hip points; make sure one isn't closer to the same-side shoulder than the other is to its shoulder, or closer to the floor than its mate.
- *Spine*. Make sure both sides of your spine are equally long.
- *Shoulders*. Make sure one shoulder isn't closer to the same-side ear than the other is to its ear.
- *Arms*. Your arms should be evenly angled away from your torso.
- *Neck and head*. Like the sides of the spine, the sides of your neck should be evenly long so your head isn't tilted to one side; and both eyes should be equidistant from the ceiling. Look at the underside of your chin; see that it's perpendicular to the floor, not pushed up toward the ceiling.

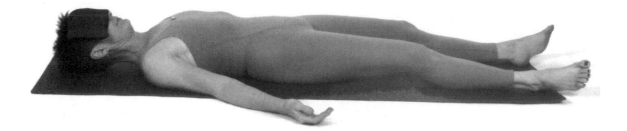

BENEFITS

Corpse quiets the body and brain and relieves stress.

CAUTION

If you have a back injury or strain, perform this pose with your knees bent over a bolster or thick roll of blankets.

TIP

To soften the groins in this pose and help quiet the body and brain, lay a 10-pound sand bag over each top thigh, parallel to the lines of the groins. Then pretend the femur heads are sinking away from the weight, toward the floor.

It's also important to stay as still as possible when practicing Corpse. Movement of any kind, even slight fidgets or nose scratches, disturbs the brain and upsets the relaxation apple cart. In addition to relaxing your physical body, also think about relaxing your "sensory body": soften the root of your tongue, the wings (alae) of your nose, and the skin on your forehead, especially over the bridge of your nose. Sink your eyes into their sockets and turn them down. Sink your brain onto the back of your skull.

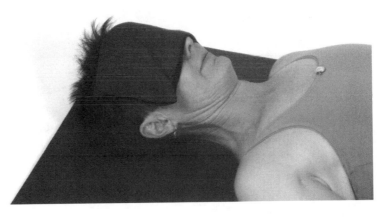

Finish both your asana and your pranayama practices in Corpse. Stay a minimum of 5 minutes, longer if you have the time.

To Come Up: Roll to your side with an exhale, wait a few breaths, then push your hands against the floor. Lift your torso with an exhale, and drag your head up like a heavy weight.

part four:

conscious breathing (pranayama)

why practice pranayama?

Pranayama is usually translated into English as "breath control." The Sanskrit word *prana* can indeed be rendered as "breath," but breath is only one manifestation of prana, which is better thought of as a subtle, all-pervasive life force or energy. *Ayama*, pranayama's second component, means to "extend and restrain." Literally, pranayama is the "extension (or expansion) and restraint of the life force."

Although pranayama has become asana's poor relation in the U.S., the practice is an indispensable prerequisite for meditation. The heart of Hatha Yoga is pranayama, not asana; it's the trigger that awakens Kundalini, our slumbering spiritual energy.

While there are hundreds of asanas, there are only a handful of pranayamas. The practice generally involves the careful regulation of *place* (in the torso where the breath is directed), *time* (or length of the inhalations and exhalations), and *number* (of breaths in a single practice session). The central technique of pranayama, called

kumbhaka (pronounced kum-BAH-kah, "pot-like"), is the purposeful stopping and retention of the breath (or more precisely, the prana) in the torso.

Several of the poses in this book are excellent preparations for pranayama: Lucky Pose stretches the thighs and hips; Bound Angle opens the groins; Twist-Around-the-Belly stretches the side ribs and belly; Bridge, supported on a block, stretches the front torso. Another important preparation for pranayama is Corpse. Be sure you're comfortable in Corpse before you begin your pranayama work.

If you want to read more about pranayama, see the Resources on page 142.

Like asana, pranayama traditionally is performed in the service of the self. But yoga also recognizes a number of physical and psychological benefits to the practice. Pranayama is said to:

- Increase the body's life energy.
- Increase the gastric fire and improve digestion

and the elimination of wastes.
- Purify the circulatory system.
- Promote mental powers (like clairvoyance) and happiness.

In this book, we'll practice pranayama for its health benefits, especially to purify our lungs and to improve our breathing mechanics and concentration.

Pranayama is usually taught in the sitting position, but most beginners have a hard time sitting "steady and comfortable," and a misaligned, fidgety body interferes with the smooth operation of the breath. Reclining, on the other hand, relaxes body tension and softens the brain, so we'll start our pranayama on our backs with our spines supported on a folded blanket.

To make such a support, you'll need two firm blankets. Fold each blanket into a long narrow rectangle measuring about 10 x 30 inches. Stack the blankets with the firm sides matching. You might also want a third folded blanket to use as a head and neck support. To use this support, sit against (but not on) the short, firm end, then lie back. Arrange yourself as you would for Corpse (page 128).

Always end your breathing practice with a few minutes in Corpse.

SECTION 1: BASIC BREATH AWARENESS

Breathing is as natural and as essential to life as eating and sleeping, but while most people appreciate a tasty meal and a good night's sleep, most of us pay very little attention—if any—to our breathing. The first step of pranayama practice is to get some idea of who we are as breathers.

There are various aspects of the breath you can focus on. Here we'll focus on just two: the "space" of the breath, and its "texture." To understand the former, first visualize your torso as a container, or as the yogis say, a pot. This container is, of course, filled with organs and stuff, but for this exercise you

have to imagine that it's completely empty. We know that when we breathe, the breath only moves into and out of our lungs, but in this exercise, imagine that the breath moves into and out of the entire torso, from the groins to your heart.

The texture of everyday breath is always somewhat uneven or rough; these breaths don't come and go smoothly, but rather in short jerks, with random quickenings or slow-downs, or periodic stops. In pranayama, the breath's texture should be smooth and even, which in turn will help calm the brain.

1. Lie on your support. *For this exercise, there's nothing to do; just observe your breathing as closely and "objectively" as possible. Notice, however, that as you watch, your breath will spontaneously begin to change on its own.*

2. Notice where in your torso your breath seems to move. *Most people find their everyday breathing fairly inhibited, mostly to an area in the mid-front of their torso.*

As you watch, does your breath seem to spread out, become more spacious? Remember, don't make happen, just let happen.

3. Notice your breath's texture. *Look for small jerks or pauses in your breath, places where it slows down or speeds up. As you watch, does your breath seem to smooth out, become silkier? Remember again, don't make happen, just let happen.*

At first, practice for 5 to 8 minutes. Gradually lengthen your practice until you can comfortably observe your breath for 10 minutes. Then you're ready to start formal pranayama.

Benefit

Breathing awareness helps to calm the brain and prepare you for pranayama and meditation.

Caution

Be sure that, as you practice, you don't become frustrated, irritated, or otherwise physically or psychologically uncomfortable or upset. If you feel any of this coming on, STOP immediately.

Tip

Be conscious not only of the movement of the breath, but also its stillness at the end of the inhale and exhale.

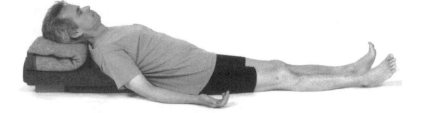

SECTION 2: PREPARATION FOR PRANAYAMA (SILENT MANTRA)

Ajapa Mantra (ah-JAHP-ah MAHN-trah)

ajapa = unspoken, silent; mantra = prayer, hymn

The Silent Mantra is "constantly and unconsciously" repeated by every breathing creature throughout its life, but the yogi should perform this mantra "consciously" (*Gheranda-Samhita* 5.90-91). Outwardly, the mantra is simply the natural sounds of the inhales and exhales, which the yogis hear as a sibilant SA and an aspirate HA, respectively (though some old texts reverse these ascriptions). It's possible, then, to make two different mantras with these syllables: SAHAM (or SOHAM), meaning "I (the individual self) am (equivalent to) She (or He or It; that is, the Great Self); or HAMSA, the Sanskrit word for "swan" or "goose," a symbol of the self ascending to the heavens (through the medium of prana, and sometimes called the *hamsa-mantra*).

The yogis learn how to amplify this sound and use it for two very practical purposes in pranayama: to absorb their consciousness in the breath, which calms the brain in preparation for meditation, and to monitor the texture, the smooth and even flow of the breath (for texture, see Section 3 below). This amplification is created by the slight contraction of the glottis, the space between the vocal cords.

1. Sit quietly for a few minutes and listen to the sound of your breath. *Can you hear the Silent Mantra?*

2. Open your mouth wide. Push your breath out of your mouth, directing as you do over the back of your throat, just behind the larynx. *Lightly* contract the base of your throat. Repeat several times.

3. Close your mouth, pressing your lips together gently. Exhale through your nostrils, and again direct the breath over the back of your throat, with the throat base lightly contracted. Inhale and take the breath in over the back of your throat. Continue to breath in this way for about 1 minute.

Caution

Be sure to contract your throat lightly. Don't overdo the mantra at first; take care that your throat doesn't become irritated.

Tip

Listen not only to the sound of the mantra, but also to the silences between the breaths, at the ends of the inhales and exhales. These short stops are natural retentions, which you'll expand later as your pranayama practice develops.

SECTION 3: BASIC PRANAYAMA BREATHING (CONQUEROR'S BREATH)

Ujjayi pranayama (oo-jie-ee)

ujjayi = to win, to be victorious, to conquer (ud = raise up; jaya = conquer)

Conqueror is the basic pranayama breath. Unlike your practice of breath awareness, where you simply observe your everyday breathing, in Conqueror you purposely alter your breathing, slowing it down (especially on the exhales), increasing its space (especially into the back torso), and smoothing it over.

I like to imagine that my inhales are rising breaths, initiated deep in the pelvis and rising to the heart (actually the subtle "yoga heart," which is in the center of the chest, a bit closer to the back torso); and that my exhales are descending breaths, from the heart to the pelvis again.

1. Lie on your support and, for a couple of minutes, observe your everyday breath. When you feel in rhythm with your breathing, consciously begin to slow it down and smooth it out. *The exhales should be somewhat longer than the inhales.*

2. Witness and listen to your mantra. Turn your eyes down and look into your yoga heart. Keep your throat soft at the end the inhale. Listen for the silences between the breaths, and make them also slightly longer (but no more than a couple of seconds).

At first, practice for 5 to 8 minutes. Gradually increase your practice time to 10 minutes.

Benefit
Conqueror prepares you for all pranayama breaths.

Caution
Pranayama is not universally accepted by all teachers or spiritually minded schools; some teachers advise against interfering with the normal rhythm of the breath. Be sure that as you practice Conqueror, your body-mind stays calm. If you feel any disturbance, STOP immediately; if the disturbance continues for more than a few weeks, consult with an experienced teacher before continuing.

Tip
To enhance your practice of Conqueror, equalize the length of your inhales and exhales. Start by counting slowly to 3 as you inhale and exhale, coordinating the movement of your breath with your count. Continue for 3 or 4 cycles, and if you're comfortable, increase the count to 4 and again continue for a few cycles. Continue increasing your count by 1 every few cycles until you find a number that suits you.

SECTION 4: BASIC SITTING FOR PRANAYAMA AND MEDITATION (EASY POSE)

Sukhasana (sue-KAHS-anna)

sukha = easy, pleasant, agreeable, gentle

Sukha is composed of two syllables: *Su* means "good, excellent, beautiful," *kha* is "cavity, hollow," and the "hole in the nave of a wheel through which the axis runs." Quite literally then, sukha means "having a good axle-hole," which at one time meant a smooth and easy wagon ride.

As with all the sitting poses, support your buttocks on a thickly folded blanket.

1. Sit in Staff (page 74). Bend your knees, cross your legs at your shins, and draw each foot toward its opposite-side hip. Rest your knees on the opposite-side foot.

2. Make sure that your pelvis is as neutral as possible; the top rim (and the perineum) should be parallel to the floor. Lay your hands, palms down, on your knees.

Begin your practice of Easy Pose by sitting for 3 to 5 minutes. Gradually lengthen your stay until you can sit comfortably for 10 minutes.

Benefit
Easy Pose is an "easy" sitting position for breathing exercises or meditation.

Caution
If you have any knee injuries, support your knees on thickly folded blankets.

Tip
If you have difficulty sitting without a back support, sit in Easy Pose with your back against a wall, or a bolster wedged between your back and the wall. Gradually try to wean yourself away from the back support.

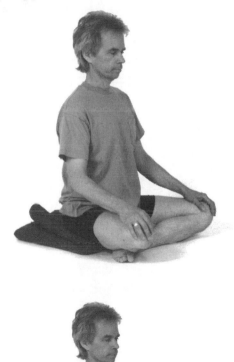

135

part five:

appendix

sequencing synopsis

It's not really worthwhile, when practicing, to perform a random series of poses. Just as you need to write letters and words in proper sequences to make your sentences comprehensible, so also do you need to orchestrate your poses and groups of poses to make the most of your practice time.

Countless sequences are possible, and different schools have their own ideas about what makes a good sequence. In general, though, a sequence should open with simple warm-ups and/or preparations (either poses or pose-based exercises), gradually rise to more challenging poses, then fall to cooling poses (classically forward bends or restorative poses) and relaxation. The sections in Part III, and the poses in each section, are arranged in a kind of mega-sequence:

- Warm-up
- Sun Salute
- Standing postures
- Belly strengtheners
- Arm strengtheners
- Back bends
- Shoulder Stand and Plow
- Twists and/or forward bends
- Cool-down
- Pranayama
- Corpse

But remember, nothing in this sequence is carved in stone. You should experiment with different types of sequences at first (e.g., Iyengar style or Desikachar style) to find the type that suits you best.

Each group of poses has its own sequencing possibilities, which allows for a lot of sequencing creativity. As a beginner, you should mostly follow the sequencing suggested here or in the instructional manuals listed on page 142. But once you acquire some practical experience, and understand the ins and outs of the poses a little better, then there's no reason why you can't devise sequences of your own.

a general how-to of sequencing

The first thing to consider when sequencing a practice is how much time you have: 30 minutes? An hour? It's rumored that Mr. Iyengar practiced more than ten hours a day when he first began teaching. Your time frame will determine how many poses you can reasonably expect to practice.

Next, every sequence needs a "hook" or organizing principle. You could, for example, sequence according to a specific body part (e.g., shoulders), or a specific group of poses (e.g., twists). Then you could sequence a medley of poses, selecting one or two from each group, so that you have a shortened version of our mega-sequence.

Rather than give you specific sequences, which get really boring after awhile, here's a general how-to of proper sequencing. Remember, though, as an Iyengar-trained teacher, I have a particular sequencing filter; be sure to expose yourself to other filters to find the sequencing grammar that's right for you.

WARM-UPS

Warm-ups can either be focused or general. In other words, you can warm up a particular area of the body (e.g., the shoulders) in preparation for a focused practice, or you can warm up the entire body for a general practice. Downward Facing Dog warms up the shoulders and opens the chest. Bent-Knee Lunge stretches the thighs and groins, and is a preparation for back bends. Reclining Big Toe stretches the backs of the legs, getting them ready for standing poses or sitting forward bends. Bound Angle stretches the hips and groins in preparation for standing poses, sitting forward bends or twists, and even back bends. Twist-around-the-Belly stretches the spine and readies the body for twists. Sun Salute is a vigorous general warm-up. Three to ten Sun Salutes will warm up the entire body quickly.

Always begin your practice with at least one warm-up.

STANDING POSES

The 11 standing poses can be sequenced in countless ways. Typically, Tree or Triangle begin the standing sequence, followed by Extended Side Angle; Revolved Triangle can be inserted between the latter two during a longer practice, or when working specifically on twists. In the Iyengar system, Warrior II usually precedes Warrior I; the latter pose should be included when preparing for back bends. Half Moon works well after either Triangle or Warrior II. Intense Side Stretch should come near the end of the sequence, after the legs are warm and stretched. Intense Wide-Leg Forward Bend and Intense Stretch can both be used either as warm-ups for the standing poses and sitting forward bends, or they can be practiced as focus poses in themselves; in addition, Intense Stretch can be used as a resting pose between individual standing poses.

Powerful Pose can be practiced anywhere in the sequence; for example, you could come out of Tree right into Powerful, or you could precede each resting Intense Stretch with Powerful.

As a beginner, your practice should concentrate on standing poses. Depending on your practice time, always perform at least two or three standing poses.

ABDOMINALS

Abdominals need consistent practice to have any benefit. Try to practice at least one abdominal every practice session.

ARM STRENGTH

Like the abdominal, the arm-strength poses need consistent practice. As a beginner, try to practice Vashishtha's Pose 2 or 3 times a week.

SITTING POSES AND FORWARD BENDS

Staff is mostly used as a ready position for the sitting forward bends and twists, but it can be practiced as a pose in itself. Hero, Cow Face, Bound Angle, and Reclining Big Toe are warm-ups for the sitting forward bends, or they can serve as focus poses; in addition, Hero and Cow Face are preparations for back bends. Head-to-Knee, Seated Wide-Leg, and Intense Stretch-of-the-West can be practiced singly, or sequenced in any way. For daily practices, sitting forward bends can be alternated with back bends.

SITTING TWISTS

Bharadvaja's Pose, Marichi's Pose, and Lord-of-the-Fishes are usually sequenced as listed. Sitting twists (as well as Chair Twist) are also good back-relief poses after sitting forward bends and back bends.

BACK BENDS

Intense Stretch-of-the-East and Serpent are warm-ups for back bends, or focus poses in themselves; in addition, Intense Stretch of the East is an arm strengthener. Locust, Bow, and Camel are usually performed as listed. Upward Facing Dog is a challenging back bend that can also be used as an arm strengthener.

SHOULDER STAND AND PLOW

Bridge is a preparation for Shoulder Stand and Plow; it's also a preparation for back bends, or it can be practiced as a back bend in itself. Shoulder Stand is what I call an "everyday pose." If you want to develop this pose, you should perform it in every practice; your short-term goal should be 3 minutes, long-term 5 minutes. By the same token, it's usually not beneficial to practice Shoulder Stand intermittently; instead, work with Modified Shoulder Stand. This latter pose is also a good cool-down pose, and a back relief after back bends and sitting forward bends.

RESTORATIVES

Inverted Action Pose is a passive alternative to Shoulder Stand. It's also a good resting pose, held for 5 to 10 minutes, after a long day of sitting, standing, or walking (or running). Child's Pose is a general resting pose; it can be used near the end of practice, or periodically during practice. Corpse should conclude EVERY practice; resist the temptation to skip over this essential pose.

how to keep the yoga fire burning

It's one thing to begin a yoga practice, quite another to keep it going. B. K. S. Iyengar says somewhere that our practice "waxes and wanes like the moon," which I've found, after nearly a quarter-century of practice, to be right on the mark. There are times when you can't wait to practice, and practice itself feels wonderful; there are other times when the last thing you want to do is practice, and practice itself feels like a visit to the dentist.

So what can you do to keep the yoga fire stoked over the long haul? Where do you find the inspiration to plug away when all you really want to do is relax and read a book? First, be sure to alter your sequencing periodically, just to keep things fresh. Treat yourself occasionally to some exercise or pose that's out of the ordinary. Don't forget that the 50 poses in this book aren't the only ones in the world. Once you've established a comfortable practice rhythm, experiment with poses from other sources, and add the ones you enjoy to your repertoire.

Don't get discouraged if things don't go well for a few practices in a row. Progress in yoga is never a straight line—it's more like a spiral, or any relationship with a significant other, sometimes loving and close, other times cool and distant. Sometimes you'll seem to be making enormous headway, other times you'll seem to be sliding downhill, like Sisyphus under the weight of his boulder. Always remember that, as Krishna counsels Arjuna in the famous *Song of the Blessed One* (*Bhagavad-Gita* 2.40, translation by Stephen Mitchell):

> On this path no effort is
> ever wasted,
>   no gain is ever reversed;
>   even a little of this practice
>   will shelter you from great
> sorrow.

Treasure the good times, but expect the hard; rest assured that every student, no matter how raw or advanced, experiences rough patches in the road. These ostensible steps backward are often a signal that significant change is right around the corner.

Always take a couple of minutes at the end of a satisfying practice to appreciate how you feel, and remember this feeling during the hard times. If you miss a day or two, shrug your shoulders and accept it, don't beat yourself over the head. Then pick up your practice again with a smile. If the hard times persist for a couple of months or more, though, get the advice of an experienced teacher.

Yoga can be a solitary occupation, so sometimes it's nice to practice with a partner, maybe a good friend or family member. Or you could organize a yoga club and meet periodically for practice; each member of the club could take a turn leading the session, or you could hire a professional teacher as a leader.

how to find a teacher

How do you find the perfect teacher? First, your local Yellow Pages will list teachers and schools in your area; look under "Yoga Instruction." Call the listed schools or individuals and ask for a schedule of classes or if they have a website. *Yoga Journal*, the most widely read yoga magazine in this country, publishes a yearly "Yoga Teachers Directory" that lists teachers state by state; the magazine also has an informative website at www.yogajournal.com. Ask your friends or office-mates to recommend a teacher or school; everyone nowadays seems to attend, or knows someone who attends, a yoga class.

Once you've gathered all your information, talk to someone at each school or, if possible, the teachers of any of the classes you're interested in. Be sure to first find out about the school's approach: some classes, like Ashtanga Vinyasa or Bikram, are notoriously vigorous, while others, like Kripalu, are milder. Be sure you have an inkling of what you're getting into

before you go, to avoid any unpleasant surprises.

You might also want to know: the length of the class and its cost; the kind of dress that's recommended; and if the school provides you with a sticky mat, or if you need to bring your own.

Begin with a beginners' class, even if you've been practicing for awhile. Most beginning classes are on-going, which means you'll be joining a more experienced group of students; some of my "beginners" have been with me for a decade. If this seems intimidating, if you have concerns about looking "foolish," remember that everybody in the room (including the teacher) was once a beginner and have nothing but good wishes for you.

If you have any physical problems or limitations, tell the teacher BEFORE class; don't surprise your teacher with a gimpy knee or a four-month pregnancy during or after class. If you're able to sample a few different teachers, try one or more classes with each one. Don't expect

miracles: if nothing seems to "happen" after the first class, don't be disheartened. Try the same teacher again, or try another teacher, or try another school, until you find the right person and environment for you.

Once you've settled on a teacher, study with that one person as much as possible, especially if you're working with a particular problem. That way the teacher will get to know you and can tailor poses and instructions to accommodate your special needs.

There are a few things to watch out for in class: NEVER perform any pose that generates "bad" pain (page 13); either tell the teacher what you're feeling and ask for an alternative pose, or simply stop altogether and rest until the next pose. Also, many teachers make manual adjustments in class. ALWAYS be sure you're comfortable with the contact: if the adjustment is too extreme, or the touch is somehow inappropriate, ask your teacher to PLEASE stop.

resources

BREATHING

Donna Farhi. *The Breathing Book*. Holt, 1996.

Gay Hendricks. *Conscious Breathing*. Bantam, 1995.

B. K. S. Iyengar. *Light on Pranayama*. Crossroad, 1981.

Dennis Lewis. *The Tao of Natural Breathing*. Mountain Wind, 1997.

Richard Rosen. *The Yoga of Breath: A Step-by-Step Guide to Pranayama*. Shambhala, 2002.

Michael Sky. *Breathing: Expanding Your Power & Energy*. Bear & Company, 1990.

Carola Speads. *Breathing: The ABC's*. Harper Colophon, 1978.

ASANA INSTRUCTION

Jean Couch. *The Runner's Yoga Book*. Rodwell, 1990.

Judith Lasater. *Relax & Renew*. Rodwell, 1995.

Elise Browning Miller. *Life Is a Stretch*. Llewellyn, 1999.

Linda Sparrowe with Patricia Walden. *The Woman's Book of Yoga & Health*. Shambhala, 2002.

Rodney Yee with Nina Zolotow. *Moving Toward Balance*. Rodale, 2004.

index

about the author

Richard Rosen recently completed the first fifty years of his life. He began his study of yoga in 1980, and has been teaching since 1987. He's a contributing editor at *Yoga Journal*, and the author of *The Yoga of Breath* (Shambhala, 2002), an introduction to pranayama. He's also working on a book about the history of yoga in the U.S. Richard lives in beautiful Berkeley, California. He wants to thank his teachers: Everything of value in this book comes from them; the mistakes are his alone.

other books by ulysses press

ASHTANGA YOGA FOR WOMEN: INVIGORATING MIND, BODY, AND SPIRIT WITH POWER YOGA
Sally Griffyn, $17.95
Presents the exciting and empowering practice of power yoga in a balanced fashion that addresses the specific needs of female practitioners.

YOGA IN FOCUS: POSTURES, SEQUENCES, AND MEDITATIONS
Jessie Chapman   photographs by Dhyan, $14.95
A beautiful celebration of yoga that's both useful for learning the techniques and inspiring in its artistic approach to presenting the body in yoga positions.

YOGA FOR PARTNERS: OVER 75 POSTURES TO DO TOGETHER
Jessie Chapman   photographs by Dhyan, $14.95
Features inspiring photos of the paired asanas. It teaches each partner how to synchronize their movements and breathing, bringing new lightness and enjoyment to any yoga practice.

YOGA THERAPIES: 45 SEQUENCES TO RELIEVE STRESS, DEPRESSION, REPETITIVE STRAIN, SPORTS INJURIES AND MORE
Jessie Chapman   photographs by Dhyan, $14.95
Filled with beautifully photographed sequences that relieve stress, release anger, relax back muscles and reverse repetitive strain injuries.

To order these books call 800-377-2542 or 510-601-8301, fax 510-601-8307, e-mail ulysses@ulysses press.com, or write to Ulysses Press, P.O. Box 3440, Berkeley, CA 94703. All retail orders are shipped free of charge. California residents must include sales tax. Allow two to three weeks for delivery.